TO Carol
This is a story of
love + faith,

House
of Miracles

Where Medicine And Miracles Meet

Cliff Fazzolari

Cliff Fazzolari

SterlingHouse Publisher, Inc.   Pittsburgh, PA

House
of Miracles

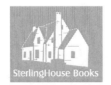

SterlingHouse Books

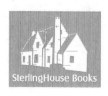

ISBN-10: 1-58501-114-2
ISBN-13: 978-1-58-501114-8
Trade Paperback
© Copyright 2007 Cliff Fazzolari
All Rights Reserved
Library of Congress #2007927167

Requests for information should be addressed to:
SterlingHouse Publisher, Inc.
7436 Washington Avenue
Pittsburgh, PA 15218
info@sterlinghousepublisher.com
www.sterlinghousepublisher.com

SterlingHouse Books
is an imprint of SterlingHouse Publisher, Inc.

SterlingHouse Publisher, Inc.
is a company of CyntoMedia Corporation.

Cover Design: Brandon M. Bittner
Original Artwork By: Brandon M. Bittner
Interior Design: Kathleen M. Gall

Printed in U.S.A.

Dedication

This book is dedicated to my boys,
Matt, Jake, and Sam—
and to the memory of Heather Cataldo
and Hunter Kelly.

Foreword

Have you ever pondered over what it would be like in this present generation if we were devoid of hospitals? Maybe that's stretching it a bit. What about the absence of specialized care for children? Most parents are very familiar with their neighborhood pediatrician, but gratefully unfamiliar with the local hospital.

Unless you have been faced with an issue requiring specialized care, the hospital is more than likely the last place you want to go. We dread going there because we are fearful of the many reasons why we might have to go to such a place. Our impression of all that is involved at a hospital is so jaded, even before we ever walk through the doors. Besides, with all the negative stories you hear in the media regarding health care, one just might think that they are actually better off not going to a hospital.

When faced with the greatest heartbreak of our lives, our family had no choice but to become very familiar with our local children's hospital—The Women and Children's Hospital of Buffalo, New York. Our initial experience began in the Department of Neurology where we were told that our infant son, Hunter, would not live past his second birthday. As a result of a very rare, degenerative, genetic disease called Krabbe Leukodystrophy, we were told to take our son home and basically wait for him to die.

There are no adequate words to describe the pain and frustration we experienced when told such devastating news. Our relationship with The Women and Children's Hospital of Buffalo began that afternoon and grew over the eight and a half years God blessed us with Hunter's life.

Relationships involve trust and respect. Over time, we learned to not only trust the experts at The Women and Children's Hospital of Buffalo but also respect them. Their respect for our family and their desire to do whatever they could to care for Hunter's needs was remarkable. Because Hunter's disease was not well known at the time, most of the physicians and nurses knew very little. Communication and patience was vital. The many experts and specialists we dealt with over the years were willing to listen—listen to us as parents and most importantly, listen to Hunter. Although Hunter never spoke a word, the doctors listened to him. They were gracious and patient enough to listen to the boy and not just treat the disease. Our confidence in the care Hunter would receive grew with our relationship. While Hunter was clearly the quarterback, it was always a team effort. Each specialist, doctor and nurse had a specific role to play and did so with confidence and compassion. No matter how knowledgeable and professional a doctor is, without compassion his or her efforts are worthless. Our "home away from home" became a place where hearts were woven into a tapestry of lifetime friendships. It was in our darkest hours that we realized how very fortunate we were to be surrounded by the outstanding Women and Children's Hospital of Buffalo team. We will not forget all that we learned through our experience and we will continue to support not only the medical team at The Women and Children's Hospital of Buffalo, but the families as well.

God has blessed our family in so many profound ways. Our lives are forever changed. We are so thankful that we have had the opportunity to witness and give testimony to the great work going on at The Women and Children's Hospital of Buffalo. The stories in this book are very real. The hope and joy experienced through immense trials and suffering are unforgettable. God has not only given us a faith that sustains us, but He has also graciously given us a haven of hope and healing through The Women and Children's Hospital of Buffalo.

—Jill Kelly

Hunter's Hope Foundation was established in 1997 by Pro Football Hall of Fame member and former Buffalo Bills Quarterback Jim Kelly and his wife, Jill, after their infant son, Hunter, was diagnosed with Krabbe Leukodystrophy, an inherited, fatal nervous system disease. The foundation is the Kellys' life-long commitment to increase public awareness of leukodystrophies as well as to increase the likelihood of early detection and treatment. Their ultimate goal is to raise money to fund research efforts to identify new treatments, therapies, and a cure for Krabbe and other leukodystrophies.

Table of Contents

Introduction

*"If the only prayer you ever say in life is "Thank you"...
that is enough."*
—*Meister Eckert*

It occurs to me that there never seems to be enough time in the day to think about the true heroes in life. In recent times, society has seemed to elevate the achievements of professional athletes and Hollywood movie stars. In a truly convoluted manner, I had a real tendency to look at life the same way. It all changed for me on October 7, 2001 when my son, Jacob, was diagnosed as having a massive tumor in his chest. For the next several weeks, my family was turned upside down as Jacob fought for survival. We were lucky; Jacob was cured and is an extremely healthy young boy. We weren't left to worry about blood tests or white blood cell counts. Instead, we were allowed to take our child home and continue our lives with him by our side. Yet, years later, there seemed to be a void in my life as I considered the men and women who banded together at The Women & Children's Hospital of Buffalo. I spent a considerable amount of time contemplating a way to thank the people who worked with us to help Jacob through his illness. I brought donuts to the ICU unit and sent baskets of fruit to his surgeons. As a family, we made a few donations, and on a daily basis we sang the praises of everyone involved, and yet, it still didn't seem to be enough. There was simply a void in my heart as I struggled to understand how the administrators, nurses, doctors, nurse practitioners, security guards, and custodians could band together to make The Women & Children's Hospital of Buffalo the first-rate institution that it is.

In the years following Jacob's illness, and as we returned to our normal routine, my inability to properly say thank-you continued to gnaw at me. Curiosity also played a big part as I wondered about the individuals who filled the uniforms. Coincidentally, I volunteered to work as part of the Family-Centered Care program implemented by the hospital staff. As a parent advisor, I found myself in a unique position in that I was now a small part of a team. Under the guidance of Women & Children's Hospital staff members, I felt as though I were really offering assistance to other families who found themselves in the unenviable position of caring for a sick child. At the same time, I came into contact with families whose children were really suffering and would never be the same. I also met the mothers and fathers who suffered through the death of their children. More than anything else, I knew I needed to do something more. I wanted to tell the story of the families and in some way, I wanted to incorporate the care they received at the hospital. I began a book featuring interviews of people associated with the hospital, but a strange thing happened as I began the interview process. Rather than this book being about my wanting to say "Thank-You", it became a tale of true heroics. The staff members and family members interviewed for this story could not understand why I wanted to speak with them. Their abilities and their heartfelt dedication did not seem like such a big deal to them. From the Women & Children's Hospital President Cheryl Klass to patients Olivia Stockmeyer and Anthony Stinson, this story became a tale of human interest and emotion. The story evolved into a piece about caring for, watching over and loving our most precious resource: our children.

In the end, I became a better person for having met the people profiled in the pages of this book. I started the project wondering how in the world I could possibly get the job done, and about halfway through I realized I was simply a typist, as one by one these stories unfolded. This is a tale about a remarkable group of people who are entrusted with the care of our children. It is a story about the human condition. It is a story about life, and a story about love. It is a way for all of us to say "Thank-You" to a small set of true heroes who work hard every day and find their own rewards in the doing of the job.

CHAPTER 1

The Story of Olivia Stockmeyer
Part I

"Children represent God's most generous gift to us."
—James Dobson

If you ever have the chance to meet Olivia Stockmeyer, the first thing you'll notice is her beautiful smile. As if her wonderful grin isn't enough, you'll also be drawn to her bright blue eyes and strawberry-blonde hair. Olivia's smile certainly brings thoughts of an angel to mind, but she is so much more than just a smile.

In the early months of 2005, a heart-wrenching sheet of paper made the rounds in and around Buffalo, New York. When looking at this single sheet of paper, my eyes were drawn to the beauty of Olivia. The words above the photo, however, explained the terror of a parent's worst nightmare: *Olivia Stockmeyer, 14-month-old daughter of Kevin and Kim Stockmeyer, and granddaughter of Michael and Jean Stockmeyer, entered The Women & Children's Hospital to receive surgery for a cleft palate on March 4th. Olivia experienced complications during that surgery and is currently in the intensive care unit at The Women & Children's Hospital in an induced coma, on a breathing machine, with serious lung problems. Your prayers and support are appreciated.*

★   ★   ★

The story of Olivia Stockmeyer is difficult to tell without first understanding the love of her parents, grandparents, and loving extended family. Late in the year of 2001, just after the terrorist attacks on New York and Washington, Kim cancelled a vacation to Las Vegas. The world was suddenly an unsteady place, and Kim wasn't real keen on traveling by air. Perhaps fate played a role, however, because, instead of being far away in Las Vegas, Kim was at happy hour in a club on Delaware Avenue. It was at this club that Kim met Kevin. Although each had graduated from Sweet Home School, they had never met until that evening. Over drinks, they formed a friendship that blossomed into a relationship that evolved into marriage. Kim and Kevin enjoyed one another's company, and before long they realized that they shared each other's vision of raising a family. The wedding took place in 2003 and the couple was immediately blessed as they awaited the arrival of Olivia in early 2004.

"It was a first pregnancy," Kim said. "Early on, I had a routine ultra-sound and there weren't any irregularities to speak of. We were so excited about everything, and we were really looking forward to becoming parents."

"We were getting the room ready, reading books about child-rearing, and just acting like first-time parents. We were nervous, but it was a good kind of nervousness, you know?" Kevin added.

Kim and Kevin, like all expectant parents, prayed for a healthy baby, but they never really considered that there might be something wrong. "It was a normal pregnancy," Kim said. Her eyes drifted a bit as she strained to remember every detail of the nine months. "Yet, when I was about seven months along, I was walking downtown and I was actually blown over by the wind and fell to the ground. I went to the hospital to be sure that everything was all right. I was fine and the baby was fine, but we discovered that it was going to be a breech birth."

"That concerned us a little bit, but we had faith," Kevin said.

"A few weeks after that," Kim said, "I thought the baby had turned to the head down position, and we were anticipating a conventional delivery, but in the final month, I went a whole day without feeling the baby move. So I called the doctor and went back to the hospital, and we learned that the baby had returned to the breech position. It was explained to me that her back was facing outward and that her legs were folded up in front of her so that she couldn't really move. A C-section was scheduled and we prayed that it would turn out all right."

The couple arrived at Sister's Hospital in Buffalo for the birthing process. They weren't exactly sure what to expect, but their nervous energy was tempered by the fact that they would soon be parents. But the birth was anything but typical.

Like so many expectant fathers before him, Kevin waited for news on the birth of his child and the health of his wife. The pediatrician who broke the difficult news to him immediately snuffed out Kevin's excitement. "You're standing there thinking, 'Please be healthy, please be healthy'," Kevin said, "and the first words out of the pediatrician's mouth are, 'I need to tell you some things'."

Kevin is an extremely thoughtful man whose easy-going demeanor serves him well in his profession as a fifth-grade teacher at Glendale Elementary School. His eyes danced with thought as he described how he felt at that very moment.

"The doctor explained that our baby had a cleft palate, possible dislocated hips, and a skin tag. My heart stuck in my throat as I listened to his words, but in my mind, I was considering that they were all things that we could deal with. I wasn't ready for such information, but I was determined to be there for Kim and to help her through the disappointing news." Kevin forced a smile as he told the story. "I mean, it wasn't the end of the world, you know? We would get through it as a family, and that's what I was thinking: We were a family now."

Kevin decided to wait to tell Kim the troublesome news. Considering his wife's feelings first, Kevin figured that it would be best to settle in, let some of the operational lethargy wear off, and then work together to digest the news. Kevin never had the chance to tell Kim. As she was coming out of the surgery, the pediatrician stopped by and addressed the new mother. "Your daughter has a few birth defects that I need to tell you about," the man said.

"I was devastated," Kim said. "I was in no position to handle such news, and I broke down as I considered that my beautiful baby had dislocated hips. I had been born with a dislocated hip, and I had to wear casts from toes to hips for six months. I didn't want that for my baby! I just wanted a healthy child."

Kim and Kevin found themselves in the unenviable position of searching for information about the condition of their child. "I wasn't even sure if I knew what a cleft palate was," Kevin said, "let alone how they would fix such a thing. All of the worst thoughts drift through your mind. You wonder if you'll have a child that is permanently disfigured. You wonder if you did anything to cause such an affliction. I don't know about Kim, but there's a feeling of guilt, almost as if I did something wrong. I asked God why, but I knew that there wouldn't be any quick answers."

Thankfully, Olivia's hips weren't dislocated; her ligaments were simply loose from her position in the womb. Yet, as Kim spent time in recovery, an infinite number of thoughts battled for space inside of her brain. How would they handle the trips to the hospital? Who would take care of their child? Would it be a lifetime of struggles or would their baby recover?

Kim and Kevin weren't sure of much, but they were sure of one thing; they would work together, and they would deal with whatever came their way. They simply had no idea how much of a struggle it would become or what a role the staff at The Women & Children's Hospital of Buffalo and, most specifically, an on-staff chaplain, would play in their lives.

CHAPTER 2

The Story of
Sister Brenda Whelan

*"When the heart weeps for what is lost,
the spirit laughs for what it has found."*
—*Sufi Aphorism*

The thought of meeting with Sister Brenda at the Women and Children's Hospital of Buffalo sent a shiver down my spine. I was actually thinking of all of the nuns I met while growing up and attending Catholic grammar school at Holy Spirit in North Collins. I was half-expecting a woman in full nun garb like Sally Field in the *Flying Nun*.

Sister Brenda greeted me at the administrative offices. Her smile was inviting and I quickly shook her hand. I appreciated the fact that she was making time for me, but that single smile put me at ease. I followed Sister Brenda to a bank of elevators, and we made small talk as we traveled toward her office.

"Excuse me for being ignorant," I said, "but what is a chaplain?"

Sister Brenda's smile grows and I couldn't help but think that it was a smile that was meant to comfort me. It is almost as though she was wrapping me in a warm blanket and ensuring me that the interview process wouldn't be troublesome or difficult. In a strange way, I already knew what her work was all about.

"Chaplains are ministers who work in the hospital. Our purpose is to help families and patients use their own faith to get through the hard days. People seek out chaplains for a variety of reasons. We're always available—24 hours a day, seven days a week. It's a wonderful job and I love what I do."

As Sister Brenda unlocked her office, I once again recalled my grammar school days. I was half-expecting a dark, dank office where my vision of Sally Field toiled in a life of chastity and poverty. Instead, I was welcomed into a bright office that was home to a half-dozen wonderful portraits of Sister Brenda's grand nieces and nephews. There was a small desk calendar with sketched images of a nun in all types of stereotypical poses. I nearly laughed out loud, considering what was running through my mind.

"There are a number of reasons why someone might seek out a chaplain. We're available to parents when their baby is ill and they're thinking about having a child baptized, blessed or dedicated. We help out families when they are concerned about an upcoming surgery or procedure and when they just need support."

Sister Brenda led me to a seat at a conference room table just off her vibrant office. "More than anything else, we are available to patients and families when they have questions and would like someone to talk to."

Sister Brenda extended a stuffed teddy bear. It was a cute, comforting bear, and she smiled as she explained that each new patient is greeted with one of the bears. "We want our patients to feel welcome. Many times moms and dads—not to mention the children—are scared out of their minds when they walk through the door. The bear is a way for us to bridge the gap through the fear and uncertainty."

We settled into chairs across from one another. Sister Brenda smiled once more, and I quickly realized I needed to ask a question or two. I was certain of one thing: I wanted to hear this remarkable woman's story. I wanted to know how she wound up as a chaplain at the Women and Children's Hospital of Buffalo. More than anything else, I wanted to understand how she handled the heartbreak that goes along with the job of tending to sick children. I told myself to hold off, realizing we would discuss the heartbreak soon enough. Little did I know we would get right down to it.

"So, what's your story?" I asked. "Tell me about your journey to this place."

It isn't the most sophisticated of questions, but it was all the prompting that Sister Brenda needed. "Before coming here, I was a kindergarten teacher, for ten years, at Annunciation School in Elma. I've been a member of the Sisters of Mercy for the past 19 years. How I ended up here is a pretty wonderful story.

"When I was teaching, I met a wonderful boy. Andy was a student of mine, and while he was in my class, he got sick. He was diagnosed with cancer and his parents came to me for support. I became a sort of link between Andy's parents, the school and the hospital. It was difficult to watch Andy as the disease took control of him, but he was just so strong, and such a wonderful boy. His parents were searching for comfort and support."

Sister Brenda's face took on a look of extreme despair and I understood how the story was going to play out. I struggled for air and waited for the words to come from her mouth.

"When Andy was sick, I was seriously considering changing careers. I loved teaching and being around the children, but I was wondering if there was something else that I was supposed to be doing. Andy passed away on October 29, 1996 and I was just devastated. After the time I spent with him, I just couldn't imagine him not being here."

I dropped my gaze away from Sister Brenda. Of course, I was trapped in the heartbreak of the story. I thought of my own boys, Matt, Jake and Sam, and the incomprehensible thought of my life without any of the three.

"What I remember most about Andy after all of these years is his funeral. When Andy was sick, he had a lot of trouble walking. The disease really took a toll on his ability to walk pain-free. Well, I stood at the back of the hearse, with the doors open. There was a soft, beautiful kids' song playing. I think it was called 'Beautiful Feet'. Anyway, I smiled through my pain because I knew Andy was walking without pain again."

Sister Brenda paused for a long moment, and I knew she was considering Andy's short life and the tremendous impact it had on her. She fought her way through the pain and offered another bright smile, but there was more heartbreak in her next sentence. "Shortly after Andy's death, I learned of another tragic story. One of my friend's sister-in-laws gave birth to twin boys. It was a most unusual birth in that one of the boys, Spencer, died the day he was born, and twelve days later his twin brother, Chance, was born. Chance died two days after his birth."

I shook my head as though I could clear the tragic story out of my mind. "So, a mother goes into the hospital expecting to bring home two boys and instead, they both pass away?"

"Yes," Sister Brenda said. "I baptized the boys for the family and after I was done, I left a short note for the pastoral care director at the hospital, saying I wanted to volunteer my services. After being a liaison for Andy, and after feeling the pain associated with the death of the twins, I just wanted to do more, you know?"

I could hardly fathom wanting to be in the direct line of such tragedy. My heart was breaking for the mother of the twins, Andy's parents, and for Sister Brenda. I set my pen down and asked the one question that needed to be answered before the rest. "How do you do it?" I asked.

"Oh, I love my job," Sister Brenda said. "Nine out of ten days I absolutely love what I do, but God rested on the 7th day, and I remind myself of that. On the dark days, I just go into that bank of elevators, don't press any buttons, and cry."

"The heartbreak has to be overwhelming," I said.

"Yes, some days, it is." Sister Brenda nodded along with me. "But sometimes something small can have a huge impact. Just a little while ago, I was in the Emergency Room. A child came in alone, and I stayed with him until his grandma arrived. I immediately connected with the boy. I greeted him with a smile and a bear, of course, and I held his hand as his grandmother discussed his case with the doctors. As it turned out, the child was going to have to stay overnight and he was dead set against doing so. The boy's grandma and the doctors were trying to make their way through to the scared child to tell him that it would be all right. Then, finally, I tried. I told the boy he would have a nice bed, and it would be okay, you know? Well, the boy looked up at me and asked so sweetly, "Can you sleep with me?" I told him I couldn't sleep with him but I would be there in the morning to check on him, and immediately he calmed down. You see, it was just a small thing, but it meant the world to the family, and I love being a part of the process that helps a child or a family."

"So I imagine that you carry a little piece of everyone with you through the day, right?"

"Certainly," Sister Brenda said. "In fact, I don't ever come to work without thinking of Andy, or the twins, or my mother, Cora, who passed away the day before I took this job. My mom used to bake cookies for Andy, and she passed away one year and one day after Andy."

Sister Brenda explained that she started work at the hospital on October 31, 1997. "I joke a lot that I'll never be out of a job because no one else wants to do what I do." Sister Brenda laughed and I laughed along with her. "But the thing is, this is a wonderful place. I feel as though I am part of a huge family of professionals who do their jobs to the best of their abilities every single day. We have 24-hour-a-day coverage, seven days a week. I work with a group of chaplains who are on-call as needed. It's a tribute to the hospital that it supports such a service for their patients, and there are a lot of people who respect what we do. From the families to the surgeons to the people on staff, we truly make a difference, and my story wouldn't be complete without the help and support of my chaplains: Betty, Janet, Kathy, Fred, Joe, and Luther. Like I've said, we are a family who happens to work together."

Sister Brenda paused for a long moment. I waited to hear more about the hospital staff and the job the chaplains are paid to do. Instead, Sister Brenda returned directly to the heart of the matter. "Truthfully, there are times when you can't not cry. Every morning I prepare for work by asking myself if I'm ready to go where I'd rather not go."

The words struck me as so profound that I struggled for something to say to validate the courage in such a statement, but Sister Brenda didn't allow me a moment to step in. "What breaks my heart more than anything else is seeing a child that is badly hurt, disfigured, or worse yet, burnt. I sit beside the parents and try to tell them that their child is the most beautiful baby in the world. It's not a lie, either. At that very moment, that child *is* the most beautiful baby in the world."

I was still struggling with the practical aspects of reporting to work every day, unsure of what waits around the corner. How is it possible to prepare yourself for the most horrific of all tragedies, and then head home at the end of the day and find enough peace to lay your head on the pillow and slip off to sleep? Almost as though she were reading my mind, Sister Brenda stepped in. "I try real hard to maintain a balance. There are some families that return or send me thank-you notes, but I have a steadfast rule: I don't step beyond the glass doors of the hospital with a family. I have to trust that when they get outside the hospital doors, there is someone to help them. The family needs to grow and to work their way through the pain, and in my heart, they are never not there."

The one question that I was prepared to bring into each of my interviews was to establish how Sister Brenda and all of her co-workers deal with the never-ending merry-go-round of patients. "It'll never end," I said. "As thrilled as you might be when a sick child is healed, there will be another to take his place. Isn't that something that tears at you?"

"Of course," Sister Brenda said. "There are days when I just want to say, enough!"

Without warning, Sister Brenda pushed away from the table and stepped into the sanctity of her office. She was back in an instant with a small, glass figurine of a pair of hands that held the angelic image of a child. Underneath the glass image are the words, *For this child I prayed.* "That's what gets me through. Isn't it beautiful?"

I held the testament to her faith in my hands and stared at the wonderful depiction of the child. It was certainly a tremendous thought, and it explained the responsibility that Sister Brenda feels, but was it enough? The power of prayer was tremendous, and hundreds of books were written on the subject. Was the story of Sister Brenda encapsulated in the children that recovered in part because of her prayers?

"Prayers aren't magic, though," Sister Brenda said, as if to caution me away from my fleeting thought. "There are times when recoveries are made and times when they're not. Sometimes the healing is in letting go."

I imagined that my face flashed a look of confusion, because Sister Brenda stepped into the void as though she needed to save me from my own thoughts. "One of the worst moments of my time here happened in the intensive care unit. A child came through the doors badly injured, and the diagnosis was quite poor. The father greeted me and demanded that I pray for his child. Of course, I was prepared to do so, and with the family and alone, I prayed—with all of my heart, I prayed. But the child didn't recover, and when I saw the father again, he confronted me. He told me that I didn't pray the right way and that the sorriest thing he ever did was to ask me to pray for his child. It simply broke my heart."

"That has to be the hardest part of your job," I said. "You have to feel as though you're surrendering."

"In a sense, you do. If I didn't believe, though, I couldn't come back every day and do what I do."

Sister Brenda paused for a moment. "As a woman in a religious community who has taken a vow of celibacy, I never expected to be present at so many births. Each one is a graced moment, a privilege. I've seen so many children enter the world in all their glory. I am reminded of the miracle of a successful birth too. It's simply wonderful."

I was beginning to understand the comfort and support of Sister Brenda. In a moment when sadness had threatened to tear me apart, she had injected a ray of sunshine. "You must feel as though you have a hundred children," I said.

"Oh yeah, hundreds! Each child is a part of me, as are many

members of the staff. In a way we are all part of a family. We laugh, cry and joke together. Julie, who is my friend first and my boss second, will often remind me when I need a kick to keep going. Julie will tell me to 'Do my best, and keep working hard'. With a friend like that, who wouldn't keep moving?"

"If I were to ask you point-blank, could you come up with a best day?" I asked.

Sister Brenda flashed a brilliant smile. I watched her eyes dance through memories that she had captured in her mind. Finally, she just shook her head. "There are just too many wonderful moments. There are so many days when I feel as though what I do is important to someone."

Yet Sister Brenda did not disappoint me. She leaned across the table and reached for the glass figurine that says *For this Child I Prayed*. "A short while ago a sixteen-year-old girl was left at the hospital by her parents. She was in for a D&C after having lost a baby, and I couldn't stand to see her completely alone. I greeted her as the doctors were helping her, and she was crying, upset about everything that had happened to her. I told her I would help her through it and I promised her I would hold her hand as long as she needed me to hold it. I pulled up a chair and I held her hand through the surgery. About half an hour later, the doctor cleared his throat and whispered, 'Sister Brenda, you can let go of her hand, she's asleep.' I told the doctor that I couldn't let go of her hand. I promised that I'd be there and I held her hand all the way through the surgery. I wanted to be there when she woke up, and I was."

"You have an unbelievable job," I said.

Sister Brenda laughed as though my wonder and awe were simply misplaced. To her, praying for a child and helping a family though a tragic time was second nature. "I'm a bit of a clown around here too," she said. "I've tried to develop a sense of humor about things, and it really helps when I'm with a sick child or a worried parent. We run the gamut of emotions around here, and sometimes it pays to be silly. Ask my co-workers: I can be as playful as anyone."

"Worst day?" I asked.

"Oh, there are a lot of those too. Anytime a family loses a child." Sister Brenda's voice trailed off and she turned the glass figurine over and over in her hand.

I felt horrible having asked the question, as I knew that I'd left her in a place where many of the memories of pain were rushing through her mind.

"One time a child passed and his parents considered having his organs harvested. What a wonderful, unselfish thing to do, right?"

I nodded as the sadness took control of my heart.

"The parents were extremely concerned about the procedure. Even in death, they were concerned for the well being of their child. I told them that I would stay with their child through the procedure, and I did. The doctors and the transplant team granted me permission, and I was able to observe the entire process. I was able to go back to those parents and tell them that their child was treated with the utmost respect, and now I can soothe the minds of other parents that are in the same position. I can tell them that I saw it happen, and I can assure them that their child will be treated with respect."

As Sister Brenda finished her story, I couldn't help but think of all of the other nuns I'd met in grammar school. I had been seriously deficient in understanding their place in the world, and in some respects I had entered the room completely unsure of the importance of the pastoral care at the Women and Children's Hospital of Buffalo.

"You can't do this job and not think of a bigger picture," Sister Brenda said. "We treat people of all different cultures and backgrounds, and I don't try to impress any of my beliefs on them. I simply try and help them find the God-given strength they have inside." Almost as though she'd been struck by an overpowering thought, Sister Brenda leaned forward. "You have to meet Father Jim Dukas," she said. "He's the Pastor at the Hellenic Orthodox Church of the Annunciation, and he does something that is just awesome." Once more, Sister Brenda's hands found the *For this Child I Prayed* figurine. "Whenever Father Dukas hears the helicopter heading for the helipad, he stops what he's doing and he prays for the child that is being transported to the hospital."

"That is beautiful," I said.

"He even stopped in the middle of mass once. He was so tuned into the sound of the helicopter that in the middle of his mass, he stopped, and asked the congregation to pray along with him."

"I see what you're saying," I said. "I can understand how you enjoy nine out of ten days here."

"I think of this place, and my life, as just a huge puzzle. I just want to be one piece that fits in someplace." As we returned to Sister Brenda's office, I couldn't help but glance at each of the photos on the wall behind her desk.

"I have 19 nieces and nephews and 23 grand nieces and nephews," she said. Sister Brenda moved to a spot on her file cabinet, picked up a bear and held it up for my inspection. "This bear was made of a table cloth that belonged to my mother."

I wasn't sure I could handle much more. Plain and simple, Sister Brenda was a testament to my faith in mankind. As with the other members of her staff, she gave more on a daily basis than most people could ever conceive of doing. My eyes drifted to a small, yellow Post-it note underneath her computer screen. Sister Brenda followed my eyes. "It says 'Kristi', she said. "Kristi is the wife of John in the public relations department. They recently adopted a child, and Kristi is pregnant. I posted Kristi's name so I remember to pray for her each day."

For this Child I Prayed.

It was an absolute pleasure to spend time with Sister Brenda. She ended our talk with yet another smile. I understood that I was a better person for having met her. I wondered how many other hundreds of people felt the same way.

CHAPTER 3

The Story of Anthony Stinson
Part I

"When you have no choice, mobilize the spirit of courage."
—*Jewish Proverb*

There wasn't a single thing in my life that prepared me to meet Anthony Stinson. My son had been very sick; there was no getting around that. I had suffered as he awaited surgery to remove the tumor in his chest. I wondered what I would do with the rest of my life if each and every one of my prayers weren't answered. Fortunately, I was one of the lucky ones. My son, Jake, made a full recovery and is free to enjoy his life. Jake spends hours jumping on the trampoline, wrestling with his brothers, and playing baseball. He runs through the house with reckless abandon and sometimes it's all I can do to keep from screaming at him to settle down and be quiet. Given Jake's renewed energy, I certainly wasn't prepared to meet Anthony Stinson.

When I arrived at the Stinson home, I was greeted with a placard on the front door that screamed: "Oxygen! No Smoking! No Open Flames! Keep Oil and Grease Away!"

I knocked lightly on the door and Anthony's mother, Trina, opened the door quickly. Upon seeing me she said, "Oh my God, I forgot you were coming." A small dog tried to escape between my legs. Trina reached for the animal and caught it. "Come on, Corabell, get in here."

I had met Trina through The Women & Children's Hospital of Buffalo's Family-Centered Care Program. I had been impressed with her dedication to the program and the fierce, protective love that she had shown when speaking about her sons, Anthony and Nicholas.

"Come in," Trina said, "but excuse me for one moment."

Trina escaped into the other room as I stood with my notebook at the ready. Before I'd made more than three steps into the home, a young boy greeted me. "Hi, I'm Nicholas," he said. "Anthony's in the living room."

I smiled at Nicholas and followed him down the short hallway that led to the living room. My heart jumped into my throat as I saw Anthony in the hospital bed in the center of the room. My eyes went directly to the oxygen bottle at the front of the bed, and then I slowly scanned the room, taking in the fully stocked medical facility that served as the family living room. Across from the bed I noticed large letters strung across the wall as if to teach a child the alphabet.

"I'm sorry," Trina said as she entered the living room. "Some days get real busy around here."

On the wall underneath the alphabet were two large chalkboards noting the minute-by-minute care necessary to sustain Anthony's life. I glanced at the medicine that needed to be administered and I even read the words of a warning posted to the nurses that assisted Trina in Anthony's care. I was doing all I could not to look into the bed.

"You've met Nicholas," Trina said, "And this is Anthony."

I peered over Trina's shoulder at Anthony as he lay in the bed. He was hooked to a number of machines, and my eyes instantly went to the trachea tube. "He's a big boy," I said.

"Yeah, he's my baby," Trina said.

"He's bigger than me," Nicholas said. "I'm two years older than him and he weighs more than me."

Trina lowered the bed rails and sat beside her unresponsive son. "Thank you for doing this," she said. "It'll do me good to talk about Anthony and the hospital."

I suddenly realized that I wasn't going to be able to just sit in the room staring at what I was seeing. I gulped for air and offered a smile. "I hope I can do your son justice," I said. My eyes returned to the wall and the note posted for the nursing staff. I couldn't help but feel the love in Trina's printed words: *Please, please, please—Always keep the side up on Anthony's bed, even if you're sitting in the chair. We take for granted that he doesn't move, but there have been a few times that, from his back, he stretched and rolled on his side. If the rail were down, he would have fallen out of his bed. One of my biggest fears is to have him fall 3 feet to the ground, not being able to catch himself. It makes me sick to think of, so please, make sure his sides are up at all times.*

"So, how do you want to do this?" Trina asked.

It dawned on me that I was just sitting there, trapped in a state of undeniable confusion. I strained for another breath of air. "How about at the beginning?" I asked.

"That would be Nicholas," Trina said. "Nicholas was born on June 23, 1998. He's a big help around here, aren't you?"

Nicholas had strayed a few feet away from the living room, but he was hanging there on the periphery to see if he could add anything about his brother. "I try to help," Nicholas said softly. "I counted all the alcohol swabs."

"Yes! You did," Trina said. She shared a brief smile with her older son. "He's a big help," She whispered. "Anthony was born on June 15, 2000, almost exactly two years later. It was a normal pregnancy, but I was a week-and-a-half early. I had gone through childbirth with Nicholas, so I figured that I knew what I was doing, but the pain was excruciating—way worse than with Nicholas. They finally administered an epidural, which was wonderful. I spent the next couple of hours pushing and joking that I wanted to name my child Anthony Epidural instead of Anthony Thomas. Yet, as it turned out, I had to have an emergency C-section."

Trina turned to the bed and adjusted Anthony's covers. "I can remember being panicked about the C-section. I was in shock actually because I had always skipped over the sections about C-sections and I felt so unprepared, but little did I know that it was just the beginning of challenges Anthony and I would face. When they finally delivered Anthony, he was screaming. I held him for the very first time, and I can remember just shaking with joy. It had been a difficult challenge, but I had my reward. I wasn't able to see Anthony for the first few hours because he was having respiratory and feeding difficulties, but when they finally got me to a room, I asked for a wheelchair because I couldn't handle being away from him." Trina gazed into the bed and a slight smile broke across her face. "Anthony had tubes and monitors hooked up to him, and that really was upsetting. I cried, but everyone said he was okay, and I was able to take him home with me."

There wasn't any doubt that Trina was replaying every second of the birth. She touched her youngest son's shoulder and reached around to softly caress the side of his unresponsive face. "The first sign of trouble occurred when Anthony was four months old. I noticed that his eyes were crossing, so I took him to the eye doctor. I'll never forget it; the ophthalmologist came out and said that Anthony could barely see. I didn't believe the guy, but later on I realized that what was happening with his brain was affecting his eyesight."

Trina is an attractive young woman whose face explodes in an expression of whatever emotion she is feeling. I immediately noticed that her dark eyes were dancing with a feeling of distress. "The day when I realized that Anthony was virtually blind was horrifying. He was in a walker and I was standing right in front of him. He must have thought that I left the room because he was yelling for me, and I was just inches from him." Trina bowed her head and then instinctively turned towards the crib. "It was devastating to me to know that he would never see. They called it cortical visual impairment and declared Anthony legally blind. What it meant to me was that he would never see anything. I don't know why, but it really bothered me that he would never see an airplane, or a sunset, or his brother."

Trina turned and checked one of Anthony's monitors. She casually touched the side of her son's face, and then her face took on an expression of hopefulness. "Being blind wasn't the worst thing in the world, though. Over the next few months, I grew used to the idea, determined to make things okay for my boys. Anthony was a big, strong boy, and he was very energetic."

"Yeah, he used to jump all over me," Nicholas said.

Trina cautioned Nicholas against interrupting, but I mentioned that it was okay with me. I wanted to hear Nicholas speak of his brother. My words of encouragement brought Nicholas closer to the bed. "Anthony was real strong," Nicholas said. "He used to knock me over."

"When Anthony was eight months old, we noticed that he was sort of leaning to one side." Trina got down off the bed, put the rail into place, and then showed me Anthony's stance from long ago. "He seemed to be in pain, and every once in awhile he'd just fall over. I was so naive, but you don't consider the worst. I thought it was an ear infection."

Trina couldn't go more than a few moments without looking at the bed. Before long, I found that I was comfortable looking at Anthony in the crib.

"He would wake up crying. He would pull at his hair, like this." Trina placed her hands on her hair at each temple. " 'Hurt Momma! Hurt Momma!' he would cry."

"We had inserts placed in his shoes to help him with his balance. God, it seems a lifetime ago."

"But, he was okay, right?" I asked. I'm sure it was a strange question to Trina, but what I meant was that he was still up and moving and responsive and curious, like a baby should be.

"He had so much spirit," Trina said. "He was so determined to make things work. That's why it's so difficult now, because I knew him before! The loss of his eyesight was tragic, but we were adapting. We got bigger books and we changed things around. He was learning and he was developing. Looking back, maybe it was just false hope, or maybe I was missing something, but I didn't have a medical degree. I was relying on his doctors, and they couldn't foresee what was about to happen."

CHAPTER 4

The Stories of Linda Eschberger & Sue Popenberg

*"Everything in life is most fundamentally a gift.
And you receive it best, and you live it best,
by holding it with very open hands."*
—Less O'Donavan

I was certain that my heart was in for a beating as I stepped off the elevator and made my way toward the Neonatal Intensive Care Unit at The Women & Children's Hospital of Buffalo. I entered the unit slowly, shocked by the brightness of the brand new unit. I passed a family waiting room equipped with a television, lockers and computers that were connected to the Internet. I took notice of the bright faces of the healthcare professionals that worked in the unit as they stared back at me from a half-wall sized plaque hanging in the main hallway. There were also bright, optimistic pictures on the wall and beautiful plants set in strategic places that screamed one word to me: Life!

I thought back to my wife's pregnancies and the successful deliveries of my boys into the world. I keenly remembered the anticipation of each delivery and the subsequent moment of elation as I saw each of my children for the first time. I can remember that one simple word entered my mind after the birth of each child: Miracle!

I stepped softly through the NICU, searching for the office

of the Nurse Manager, Linda Eschberger. The words *life* and *miracle* were ricocheting around in my mind, but truth be told, I was a little nervous, as I wasn't too keen on seeing a critically-ill newborn. I knew that observing a very sick child was most likely a part of my near future.

"Hello!" Linda said as I sheepishly entered her office. She guided me to a chair across the desk from her. Although I had met Linda when my own child was sick, I was still struck by the fact that she looked too young to be in charge of such a critical unit. Yet, I was soon to find out that Linda's youthful look was made up of energy and enthusiasm. She had worked in the unit for 25 years!

"I've asked one of our critical care nurses, Sue Popenberg, to join us today," Linda said. "This is a total team effort. We've both been here forever and we're still so proud to tell people where we work."

I nodded a hello in Sue's direction and she smiled. Sue seemed to be a little uneasy about the interview, almost as though she wondered why I might want to interview her about a job she loved so much.

"Sue, how long have you been a part of the hospital?"

"Thirty-two years," she answered. "I've done everything. I've been a staff nurse, in home care, and a NICU nurse. I also assist in the research department."

I was thrown off course a bit by the fact that Sue and Linda had spent so many years as a part of The Women & Children's Hospital of Buffalo. It was almost as if they had found the fountain of youth. They both looked too young to have such experience.

"What keeps you here?" I asked.

"There are so many beautiful families," Sue said. "Meeting such wonderful people who truly love their children is all I need to make the job worthwhile." Sue's eyes instantly filled with tears. I had established a new personal record; I had brought tears to the eyes of a professional with just two simple questions!

"I can't help but think of Francesca," Sue said. She glanced at Linda, who offered an ear-to-ear smile. "Francesca was seizing in the very first twenty-four hours of her life. It's amazing, but when that happens sometimes there is a sense of resentment in the parents of the child, but Francesca was blessed with an amazing set of parents who had an unbelievably positive attitude from the very first moment. Francesca's parents didn't look around for someone to blame. Instead, through strength and faith, they just loved their daughter. It was impossible not to share their excitement for life. They were simply thrilled to have Francesca, and nothing else mattered. They considered her a miracle from the start."

It struck me that just seven minutes into the interview I had been subjected to the two words that had been smashing around in my mind as I entered the unit: Life and Miracle. Yet I was afraid to ask the question. Sue answered it before it fully formed in my mind.

"Francesca is eight years old now. The doctors have performed about ten brain surgeries on her since the day she was born, and you know what? Her family is still so strong. No matter what has happened to her, they only show us the love they feel for each other." Sue wiped at the tears in her eyes. It was a subtle flip of her hand that let me in on the secret that she knew how to be both emotional and strong. "Francesca was recently in the unit, and we were all so thrilled to see her again. At such a time we are reassured that life is good and that families are strong."

"You need that lesson over and over again, I imagine," I said. I was speaking of the difficulty of being around sick children on a daily basis, but Sue's answer surprised me.

"If you don't meet the strong parents to re-establish your faith in humanity, you'll see a lot of examples of the downside of life. Unfortunately, sometimes we have to hand children over to parents who will not care for them properly."

"It must be physically difficult to hand the children over," I said.

"Certainly," Linda answered. "Some of the children have been here for six, seven, or nine months and we've cared for them every minute of every day, and we're sort of forced to hand them to a family that doesn't have the resources, the knowledge, or the understanding to take good care of them."

The conversation lagged a moment as we all realized there was no easy answer to such a dilemma.

"Tell him about Matthew," Linda said.

Sue's eyes lit up. "In 2004, Matthew was born two and a half months premature with a congenital birth defect diagnosed as a Diaphragmatic Hernia. This is a serious condition, and Matthew underwent surgery. There were so many ups and downs that the entire unit was on a maddening roller coaster ride of emotions. Matthew was here from October through January, and I can remember crying every day through that time."

I couldn't imagine having such a challenging or demanding profession, but I didn't step in to interrupt the story.

"What was truly amazing to all of us was the love of Matthew's parents. One of the best days around here was when Michael and Charlene held Matthew for the very first time."

"Matthew is doing well?" I asked.

"Certainly. He'll be two in October and there are challenges ahead of them, but the family is just so thrilled. Their love is what makes this unit go."

Linda paged through a folder on her very organized desk and slipped a press release to me. It chronicled a benefit called *A September to Remember*. Matthew's parents organized the benefit and, in the well-written release Matthew Ruiz documented the love that Sue and Linda were speaking about.

"If someone had asked me a year ago about the Neonatal Intensive Care Unit (NICU) at Women and Children's Hospital of Buffalo, I would not have been able to provide any insight about the Unit or the miracles they perform there each day.

My wife Charlene and I were waiting to become parents for the first time—decorating our baby's nursery, preparing for the baby shower, and basically doing what expectant parents do—when suddenly our lives changed forever. On October 12, 2004, our son Matthew was born 2 ½ months premature with a congenital birth defect diagnosed as a Diaphragmatic Hernia. This condition occurs in approximately one in every 2500 births.

As Charlene and I came to grips with the severity of Matthew's con-

dition, we were amazed by the support and compassion we received from the staff of the NICU. As each day went by, we became more comfortable and knowledgeable due to our interaction with the doctors and nurses. Matthew underwent two surgical procedures before he was three weeks old, and then another surgery at two months. It was an incredible ordeal, but I am proud to say that after almost three months in the hospital, Matthew is home now and healthy. We cannot begin to express our thanks and appreciation to the staff at the Neonatal Intensive Care Unit.

With this in mind, Charlene and I want to express our gratitude and raise awareness about the incredible work done in the NICU each and every day. On September 9, 2005, we will host a black-tie charity gala and auction to benefit the Neonatal Intensive Care Unit at Women and Children's Hospital of Buffalo. The event will be held at Shanghai Red's and will offer incredible entertainment, specialty foods and an auction of unique items that will ultimately raise significant dollars for this great cause. Any monetary contribution or a donation of goods and services will directly benefit the NICU and its staff. Please join us in support of this important and worthwhile cause by attending the event or making a contribution. We will appreciate your support.

Thank you, Michael Ruiz, Chair, A September to Remember

"That's wonderful," I said. "You've touched so many families."

"It's funny, but in the time I've been here there have been so many difficult days, but we're able to get through it because we are such a team. Everyone helps out, from the nurses to the nurses aides through the custodial and secretarial departments," Linda said.

"We all pull together," Sue said. "Most of the people here love their job, and together we'll celebrate birthdays, anniversaries, and marriages."

"A celebration of life," I said.

"Exactly," Linda answered.

I hated to ask the question, as the mood in the room was upbeat. Together we were discussing all of the positive aspects of a job that had to have its moments of heartbreak and devastation. Yet, we were dancing around the raw pain that was also a very real aspect of life. "Obviously," I sheepishly began, "there are children who don't go home."

Almost on cue, Sue and Linda's eyes changed expression. Instantly, the traces of tears returned. "It's horrible," Linda softly said. "You just feel so much for the family."

"It breaks my heart," Sue said. "We'll go to the funeral and try to help the family, but it hurts so much. We put together photos and a memory book for the parents, but it's all so hard to do."

"We take the baby to the morgue," Linda said. "And I hate that because it always seems so cold there. I don't know why."

Linda looked to Sue, who shuddered as though she were actually visiting the one place where every nurse hated to go. "We dress the baby for the parents to hold and that's difficult too," Sue said. "And yes, it is a long, cold trip, but in the end, it sort of helps. I know what Linda is saying though, because I'm always trying to keep the baby warm, even in death."

"I put an extra blanket on them," Linda said.

I considered the fact that the two women before me had long accepted this difficult aspect of the job. Yet, accepting the circumstances and being able to bury the hurt were two separate things.

"How do you accept death as a part of your job?" I asked.

"I ask myself why," Linda said. "I wonder why God would do this, but He must have a purpose and we aren't real sure what it is. We band together, though. The mood on the floor is obviously down, but we all comfort the nurse or the team of people who was caring for the child. We laugh together and unfortunately, we cry together too."

"You must feel that becoming a nurse was your life's calling," I said.

"It's even more than that," Sue said. "There are different kinds of nurses, and we all seem to find a niche as a calling. I feel comfortable in the NICU, but it takes a different kind of nurse to be in the PICU. We all seem to land where we are supposed to be. One thing I do know is that seeing sick children has definitely made me appreciate what I have at home."

"Tell me about that," I said.

"I've been married to Ray for 30 years and I have four children, Kristin, Jim, Kate and Kerry. They're all doing very well and I thank God every day they've been healthy."

"How about your best day?" I asked. It was a simple question that seemed to lift the veil of despair brought about by speaking of the worst possible day. It was also a question that brought relief to Sue's eyes.

"That's easy," she said. "When the babies go home," Linda explained. "Some of the children spend months with us, and there comes a moment when they are able to go home. We dress them in their own clothes and place them in their own car seats. The parents are so excited that it is just contagious. We feel as though we've done our job."

"The parents are excited and a little scared," Linda said. "There are so many who ask us to come home with them to help them care for their child. We wish that we could."

I couldn't help but think about the personal touch of the unit. Prior to the interview, I had paged through a cut sheet of information about the Neonatal Intensive Care Unit. Reading the page had left me feeling a little distant as to what happened in the department on a daily basis. Re-reading it with Linda and Sue's voices echoing in my mind changed my perspective.

Locally unique to Women & Children's Hospital is the region's largest and most advanced Neonatal Intensive Care Unit (NICU), providing the highest level of care possible for the most critically ill newborns. As the Regional Perinatal Center for Western New York, seventeen hospitals from the region's eight counties and three institutions in Erie and Warren, Pennsylvania transfer their most critically ill infants and high risk expectant mothers to Women & Children's Hospital for this highest of skilled medical care. The teams of specialists in the Neonatal Intensive Care Unit represent highly trained and specialized health professionals dedicated to delivering the most state-of-the-art care available. Physicians, nurses, nurse practitioners, respiratory, occupational, physical therapists, neonatal transport teams, nutritionists, psychologists, social workers and pharmacists are all part of this specialized team, and are each specially trained in the care of infants and children. Critically ill newborns also

have immediate access to a complete range of pediatric sub-specialists.
Women & Children's Hospital is also the only hospital in the region to
have pediatric surgical sub-specialists for dental medicine, neurosurgery,
ophthalmology, orthopedics, otolaryngology, and urology and general
pediatric surgery. Annually, the Neonatal Intensive Care Unit cares for
more than 700 infants, nearly 300 of whom are transferred from hospi-
tals within the regional perinatal network.

"I bet you love holding children," I said.

Sue laughed. "You could say that. It's amazing, but just to touch
them sometimes makes it all worthwhile. When I started here we
didn't even have the right instruments to care for children."

"Remember," Linda said, "back in the day when a child was
less than 1000 grams we would just try and keep them comfortable. We used to work so hard just to help a child survive and
now, with technology so advanced, we are working on quality of
life. We are part of a research team that tries to educate families."

"Tell me about some of your studies," I said.

"Oh, there are so many," Linda said. "For instance, Infrasurf
is a medication developed by Dr. Egan. Infrasurf is used for the
prevention of Respiratory Distress Syndrome in premature
infants at high risk for RDS and for the rescue of premature
infants who develop RDS. Doctor Egan did a remarkable job, but
as a unit we are proud that we worked together on the study."

"The studies are almost too numerous to mention. We are
working with the neurology department on a shaken baby syndrome study." Linda glanced at Sue.

"The eye study," Sue said.

I smiled, and Sue looked at me quizzically. "Do you know
that you two often finish each other's sentences?" I asked.

"That's the way it is around here," Linda responded. "We are
truly a team."

I was certainly convinced. I was more than satisfied in the
realization that the way to capture what happened in the
Neonatal Intensive Care Unit was to speak of the team concept.

"Would you like to walk through the unit?" Linda asked.

I thought about my fear of seeing a critically-ill newborn. I wasn't quite sure that I was man enough to handle it, but Sue and Linda had provided me with a healthy perspective. I thought of how Sue's eyes lit up when I asked her if she liked to hold a child. If these two remarkable women could face it on a day-to-day basis, perhaps I was also tough enough to handle a simple walk through the unit. It still wasn't easy.

Linda escorted me through the beautiful, well-lit unit. She opened the door to a comfortable room with a couch, a rocking chair, a television and a few magazines. "We have three rooms setup so that families can stay overnight. We also have a comforting room where we can meet with a family to discuss end-of-life care."

I fought for air, as I understood that there should never have to be a room for such a service. Linda smiled through the pain of showing me such a room as I searched for something to say.

"Those are wonderful beds," I said.

Linda led me to the edge of one of the beds. "These are the Cadillac of beds for premature children," she said. "They're called Giraffe Omni-beds, and this is exactly what we were talking about when we explained how life has changed for the nurses and the patients. These beds make it so much easier to care for the child."

As I edged closer to the bed, I became aware that there was a newborn resting inside. This was the absolute moment of truth. I felt my heart rise into my throat and Linda led me to the front of the bed. I stared down at a handwritten sign that said, 'Susan— 25 weeks.' The small sign was decorated with flowers and bright colors. It was impossible not to think of the words 'miracle' and 'life.' At the same time, I contemplated the heartbreak associated with what might happen to the child. Yet I worked up the nerve to look through the glass covering over the child's head. I must have made a sound as I struggled to control my emotion. It was a sound that I'd never made before; it was a half-giggle, half-sob kind of sound that captured all that I was feeling. Linda placed a hand on my left arm. "Susan is doing great," she said. "She's going to be just fine."

As long as I live, I will never forget what it felt like to look at baby Susan. I was at a loss to explain it all to Linda at that precise moment, but her bright smile made my heart jump in my chest. Here was a tiny, tiny baby struggling to survive in a brand-new environment. It was a child that wasn't quite ready for the new world, but one that would survive with a quality of life that was dependent upon a team of professionals that loved their jobs, finished one another's sentences, celebrated marriages and births, cried together, and loved one another.

"Susan's a miracle," I whispered as I choked back tears.

"Isn't she beautiful?" Linda asked. "We're so proud of how she's doing."

I shook hands with Linda and Sue. They thanked me for talking to them about their jobs and I thanked them for doing what they do. I'm not quite sure they understood how awe-struck I was, but I headed toward the elevators with my faith in life renewed. Beautiful baby Susan would be forever in my mind. For the first time, I understood how this team made it through the merry-go-round of critically ill newborns. It was all about the miracle of life.

CHAPTER 5

The Story of Olivia Stockmeyer
Part II

"The soul is healed by being with children."
—*Fyodor Dostoevsky*

The birth of a child has very often been described as a miracle. Since the beginning of time, mothers and fathers everywhere have wanted to stand up and scream: My child was born today! The feelings are oftentimes overwhelming, and the joy is validated in the very holding of the child. The world seems to spin a little differently when you are holding a baby in your arms, and for Kevin and Kim Stockmeyer, the birth of their beautiful daughter, Olivia, was everything that they could have imagined. Yet, their enthusiasm was somewhat tempered by the fact that Olivia was struggling with "a few birth defects."

Kevin and Kim's jobs allowed them a certain receptivity in handling Olivia's difficulties. Kevin relied on his ability to organize his thoughts and attack the problem. These instincts served him well as a schoolteacher who planned daily lessons. Kim was more direct and precise in her approach, a tact that she had long ago learned as an accountant handling the complexities of corporate tax law. Kim and Kevin were certainly a good team, and Olivia proved to be in excellent hands. The first order of business was to learn about what their child was facing and to handle the problems one-by-one.

During the first year of Olivia's life, adjustments were made. Due to her position in the womb, Olivia's leg ligaments had stretched and needed time to heal. Olivia wore three diapers for those early days, but the concern over her hips subsided as Olivia grew. The true cause of concern was the cleft palate reconstruction that was necessary.

Unless you have a child that is born with a cleft palate defect you would be hard-pressed to understand that the incidence of clefting is high. It is estimated that clefting difficulties present themselves in 1 of every 700 births. Kevin and Kim's initial angst about being the cause of Olivia's cleft palate was unfounded, as there did not appear to be a genetic reason for Olivia's affliction. Through research, the proud parents discovered that Olivia's face began to form between the 4th and 8th weeks of pregnancy. In the development stage the baby's lip and palate form separately, with the lip forming first and the palate forming a few weeks after. Perhaps the position of Olivia in the womb caused her mouth to remain open and unconnected, resulting in the split or divides in her palate. In any regard, the Stockmeyer's decided to concentrate on what was necessary to correct the defect. There was no getting around the fact that Olivia was facing soft palate reconstruction surgery, but an organized approach to the problem all but assured Kim and Kevin that Olivia would be just fine.

"The first year of Olivia's life was pretty ordinary after all," Kim explained. "Olivia couldn't be nursed in a normal fashion, but she was on regular formula, and we used the Medela Haberman Feeder to nurse her. Olivia was healthy. She gained weight and was so beautiful that we nearly forgot that there was anything wrong."

The Medela Haberman Feeder is a specialized feeder that has a slit valve in the mouthpiece, which opens when the baby applies pressure. The special feeding device allowed the Stockmeyer's to nurse Olivia without too much difficulty.

"Yet the upcoming surgery was right there in the back of our minds," Kevin said. "When she was three months old, Olivia had ear tubes implanted at The Women & Children's Hospital of Buffalo by Dr. Pizzuto. We were told that she was more susceptible to ear infections, but she surprised all of us and was rarely sick. We got lucky; Olivia was a healthy, happy baby."

The Stockmeyers consulted with the staff at The Women & Children's Hospital of Buffalo and the soft palate reconstruction was scheduled to take place on March 3rd, 2005, thirteen-months after Olivia's birth. The anxious parents appreciated the team approach to the cleft palate repair as the procedure was fully explained.

"It was explained to us that making repairs to the soft palate too early could impair facial growth. If Olivia's palate was reconstructed too late, it was possible that her speech could be affected," Kim explained. "We were anxious, but we were reassured every step of the way that it was a fairly routine surgery that would return Olivia to us with 100 percent normal functioning and a completely normal appearance."

"I was worried about Kim," Kevin said. "I was real confident that the surgery would go well, but you know how anxious a mother can be. It sounds strange, but I was more concerned about how the surgery would affect us. Basically it was oral surgery, not too much to worry about, but there isn't a parent in the world that wants to see their children go through any type of procedure. And there isn't a husband in a world that wants to live with an over-anxious wife."

The true angst in regard to the surgery settled around how the Stockmeyer's were going to handle the recovery process. "Olivia wasn't going to be able to eat solid food for two weeks," Kim explained. "We were going to have to feed her using a cup, and we would have to restrain her arms. That's a pretty tall order for a baby, but we would handle it."

Kim and Kevin looked at one another and smiled. "It was sort of silly to be worried about that given what happened," Kevin said. "I really wasn't worried," he added as his voice trailed off.

Despite his insistence that everything would be just fine, two nights before the scheduled surgery, Kevin was having a difficult time sleeping. As he tossed and turned in bed, Kim grew tired of the endless flip-flopping.

"Are you going to go to sleep?" Kim asked.

"I'm trying to," the ever-practical teacher explained, "but I can't shake the feeling that something is going to go wrong. Something isn't right."

It was Kim's turn to reassure her husband. "It'll be fine," she said. "In a couple of weeks, Olivia will be good as new and we'll forget how anxious we were. Now go to sleep!"

Kevin lay in the bed staring at the ceiling. Perhaps Kim was right; maybe he was over-thinking all of it. He struggled with his feelings of apprehension until sleep took control, but when he woke in the morning, the anxiety had not quite faded. Kevin battled his instincts, but deep down, he understood that something wasn't quite right. In the day preceding the surgery, the Stockmeyers held their child just a little bit tighter.

On the morning of the surgery, Kim and Kevin set aside their anxious feelings. They had been meeting with the plastic surgeon, Dr. Shirley Anian, and Dr. Pizzuto. They had every confidence that the operation would be successful. Yet there was the idea that their child would be on an operating room table where they could not attend to Olivia's every need. "You feel real helpless, but you have to trust the team of people working on your child," Kim said. "Still, it isn't easy to take. I don't care what sort of operation it is; there's a great deal of anxiety."

There was also Kevin's feeling that something wasn't quite right.

"I started crying when the nurse came for Olivia," Kim said. "Kevin and my dad were waiting with me in the surgical waiting room, and it was all so difficult to comprehend. I had passed by the PICU waiting room, and I had thought about how horrible it would be to sit in such a room and wait for news about a critically-ill child. Olivia was screaming and crying too. The surgery started between 8:30 and 9:00 am and we sat in the room, waiting for the good news to come."

Dr. Pizzuto was the first to address the anxious parents. "It was a great relief when we saw Dr. Pizzuto. He explained that the tubes had been inserted without a problem and that we would hear from the others involved in just a short while. Dr. Anian soon followed and explained that Olivia had done fine, but that the cleft had been very wide. We were informed that Olivia might very well need additional work if she sounded nasal when she spoke, but that the second procedure was a long way off, perhaps when Olivia was about five years old."

Kim and Kevin were pleased with the information. A sweet wave of relief washed over the happy parents as they waited out the next step. "The anesthesiologist will be out to meet with you shortly," Dr. Anian explained. It was just a bit after 10 o'clock.

The minutes moved like hours as Kim and Kevin waited for news from the anesthesiologist. "Initially, we didn't really have any idea that there was a problem," Kevin said. "We were satisfied that the team had been able to do their work, and we talked about the need for the second procedure, but most of all, we were simply waiting for the moment when we could see Olivia."

Kevin's sixth sense about something being not quite right did not present itself until nearly 11:30 a.m. when the anesthesiologist entered the doors of the surgical waiting room. "We're having some slight difficulty in maintaining Olivia's oxygen levels," he said. "We're going to do a chest X-ray to find out why she's having this problem. Hopefully, it will subside and you won't have to see me again."

"It's hard to explain what we were feeling," Kevin said. "For the first time there was a palpable fear. It's almost as though you're sitting there thinking, 'This can't happen, this can't happen' as you realize that this is happening."

Inside, Kim was an emotional wreck as they waited for more news. Yet Kim and Kevin both wore brave faces. Unfortunately, the couple saw the anesthesiologist again. "Olivia has pulmonary edema, which is swelling and fluid accumulation in the lungs."

"My legs turned to jelly," Kim said. "The entire room seemed to spin as my mind tried to handle the news. I wanted to ask a hundred-and-one questions, but I was simply too stunned to verbalize it."

"We were waiting for the anesthesiologist to tell us what to do," Kevin said. "Before we reached the state of absolute panic, he explained that we could see Olivia."

"You're walking down the hall," Kim said, "but its not as if you're really moving as you've moved all of your life. I felt like my legs weighed a ton, and although I couldn't wait to see my baby, I was almost afraid of getting there."

Kim's fears were realized when she saw Olivia in the recovery room. "Her skin was a light shade of purple," Kim said. "I focused on the dried blood on her lips and it was just too much. Usually when you cry, you can feel it coming on you, but I had no warning. A sob rocked my body and I turned to Kevin to see that he was crying too. It was like a movie. It just couldn't be happening to us."

"Lynn, the recovery nurse, started to tear up when she saw our reaction," Kevin said. "I couldn't stop looking at the oxygen mask. It sort of drifted through my mind that my daughter shouldn't have to be wearing an oxygen mask! Not ever!"

Olivia, meanwhile, wasn't happy with anything that was happening to her. The beautiful, fiery redhead was letting everyone know that she didn't much care for the oxygen mask either.

"Perhaps she'll calm down if you'll hold her," Lynn said to Kim.

In the span of the two hours that seemed to pass like a month, they were the sweetest words that Kim had heard. Anxiously, she prepared herself to hold her daughter. In her heart, all that mattered was the feeling of Olivia in her arms.

CHAPTER 6

The Story of Brian Smistek

"There are only two ways to live…
one is as though nothing is a miracle…
the other is as if everything is."
—*Albert Einstein*

There are so many people that we all cross paths with on a daily basis. In many cases, the faces look familiar but we can't quite place the name. Once in a while, we have the pleasure of meeting a man or a woman who makes such a strong impression that we can never forget who they are or what they do. Parents, children, and staff members all say the same thing about Women & Children's Hospital of Buffalo's on-staff photographer, Brian Smistek. It isn't just the true professionalism of his work; that is secondary. It's not just his bright smile and eternally optimistic attitude; that also pales in comparison to his true strength: his love for others.

I had the good fortune of meeting Brian Smistek as my child was suffering through the initial stages of being diagnosed with his life-threatening tumor. I met Brian quite by accident, however, as I stopped him on the first floor hall to ask him where a particular room was in the hospital. I can remember feeling quite anxious and highly panicked as I considered my son's predicament. I had stopped Brian because he was flawlessly dressed and was already smiling when I came up to him. Out of the sheer frustration of being lost and not knowing quite where I was supposed to be, I asked Brian if he could direct me to the CT-Imaging area. "I can do better than that," Brian said. "I'll walk you there."

I had no way of knowing that Brian was just doing what came natural to him. I had no idea that the beauty of his single gesture was simply the way that Brian lived his life, but as we rode up on the elevator after meeting for the very first time, I can remember thinking, 'This is a good guy. He went out of his way to help me.'

Nearly five years later, I met Brian in his office on the 10th floor of The Women & Children's Hospital. In the years since Jacob's successful treatment at the hospital, Brian and I had become fast friends, trading e-mails and greeting each other enthusiastically on the occasions that we met. Of course, Brian has a tendency to greet everyone with the same sense of optimism. Yet he had a way of making me feel that I mattered to him, and of course, it was because I do. You see, Brian Smistek loves life and he adores human contact. I couldn't help but glance at the wall of thank-you cards that Brian had accumulated through the years. I stopped long enough to read one such card: *"Dear Brian, Thank you so much for putting together the video with all of Ellie's TV debuts! I can't tell you how much we appreciate this and all the nice things you have done for Ellie and our family—we have such beautiful pictures of Ellie & Mare—we get so many compliments on them! You are a very talented and thoughtful person and I just wanted you to know you are appreciated. Thanks Again!"*

"I like to hang up the cards because I get a thrill out of being honored for just being human," Brian said. "I take photos of sick children and present them to their parents. I love the happy looks on the faces of the families when I take the time to send them home with something."

I glanced around the room and took in each of the small faces staring back at me. It wasn't that Brian was simply being human; he was also a world-class photographer. "Tell me about how you arrived here at the hospital," I said.

Brian smiled and I could almost see the wheels turning in his mind as he thought back over the past 35 years.

"I arrived here in November of 1971," he said. "Within a week of coming here, I knew that this is where I belonged."

"What made you so sure?" I asked.

"It's about human contact, buddy. I feel such a strong connection with almost every child or family. Every single kid that walks through those doors is special to me just because of who they are." Brian guided me to his studio. He sat at his computer desk and reached down to a small refrigerator. He handed me a soda and smiled as he did so. "Look around," he said. "Over the years, I've been able to accumulate small things that make children smile. That is just so cool to me."

I sipped the soda as I followed Brian's eyes around the room. There were a few boxes of toys and stuffed animals. I saw green and gold pinwheels, photos of Winnie the Pooh and Tigger. There were also a number of beautiful photographs posted on the walls. "When you talk about human contact," I said, "I imagine that you are also speaking about the difficult days. How do you handle the endless parade of sick children coming through those doors?"

Brian smiled heavily, but his answer came quickly. "I cry," he said. "I cry all the time, but if that ever stops then I won't work here anymore."

I let the answer sink in as I scanned the walls of the studio. "Your work is magnificent," I said.

"Thank you, I appreciate that," Brian answered, "but it's about so much more than taking pictures. I take portraits of chronically ill children, dying children, children who are victims of child abuse or sexual abuse, and I have to take autopsy photos. Sometimes my heart breaks and sometimes I'm on cloud nine with happiness, but not a day goes by when I don't feel that human connection."

"You're always smiling, though," I said. "When I think back to when my child was sick, I can remember looking forward to seeing you because you always had a smile for us."

"I was born with an endless amount of smiles," Brian said, and as if to show it, he offered me one more.

"And yet, there are the child abuse cases," I said. "There has to be anger there, right?"

"Anger? No, I'm not naïve enough to think it will ever stop, but there isn't a lot of anger. Certainly I'm disappointed, but I still see the child through the pain, and I know that I can't allow them to see anger. My job is to show them happiness even if it's just for the few minutes that I might spend with them. Of course, some of the things I see are difficult to ignore or forget. There aren't a lot of people in my life who I choose to burden with these unpleasant experiences, but I get through those sad moments."

"You cry, right?"

"Yes, I cry! I cried in a patient's room just a couple of days ago." Brian glanced at a folder on his desk. I could see the angelic face of a young girl staring back at us, but I didn't want to know the details of what made such an optimistic man break into tears.

"I can't even tell you how bad I feel for that child and her family," Brian said. He leaned forward in the chair and his eyes filled with tears. "I left her room and I went straight to Target. I bought that girl some back-to-school clothes, pens, paper, glitter, a hand-held game and a few rolls of film. She's only thirteen but thinks like a thirty-year-old. I wanted her to have some things that were age appropriate, things that were meant just for her. She really wants to be a photographer and I wanted to get her started. I even gave her one of my cameras, and it made her so happy. I don't care, it was a great camera, but it didn't mean as much to me as seeing her happy, even just for a split-second."

Brian paused for so long that I wondered if he'd even go on. He sipped his soda and stared at the folder as though he could transmit healing powers through the photograph of the young girl. "I swear, Cliff, if I had a million dollars, I'd give it to her so that she never had to want for anything again."

Right before my eyes, I was watching Brian cope with the hurt that came with doing his job. I knew that I wasn't in a position to truly understand, but I also knew that Brian had a built-in support team right there at the hospital. "A lot of staff has spoken about the team concept and the wonderful support here at the hospital," I said.

"Oh my God," Brian said. "That's what it's all about, brother. We all go out of our way to help each other. If I'm here at six in the morning and the cleaning crew hasn't cleaned the elevator yet, I'll stop the elevator and clean the floor, and I'm not the only one doing things like that. We all want this place to be clean, comfortable and compassionate, and we all work together and help each other through the difficult days.

"We've spoken about the good days and the bad days. It must be a roller-coaster of emotions for you."

"Certainly," Brian said. Once more I watched his eyes change expression as he flipped through the stories captured in his mind. "You know, I think of Jessica a lot. It's so hard to pick just one child out, but you asked about the highs and lows of working here. About ten years ago there were a number of children working to help design a hospital necktie. We wanted to capture the event, and so I headed to the activity room with my camera in tow. I was there to take photos of all that was going on, but when I walked in the room, I saw Jessica. She was between four and five years old and I knew that not only was she very sick, but that she was awfully down about it too. Jessica wasn't playing with the other children. Instead, she was sitting off to the side with her mother, looking down at a blank piece of paper. Jessica was completely bald and I instantly knew that the chemo had really played havoc on her spirits." Brian closed his eyes and leaned back in the chair.

I understood that Brian was no longer doing my interview. Instead, he was back in that room, kneeling down before Jessica. "'Do you want me to help you draw something?' I whispered. Jessie had these beautiful eyes that were full of expression, and I could see that she was scared. Yet suddenly she smiled. 'Barney,' she said.

Brian's eyes remained closed but a smile broke across his face as he remembered their work. "We worked on a tie-design for a contest that would be broadcast on WKBW-TV. We laughed a lot, and Jessie's Mom whispered to me that she appreciated that I was making Jessie laugh and talk."

Brian opened his eyes and his smile faded away. "Jessica died on the morning that the winners were chosen. She never knew that her tie-design won first place."

"Oh God," I whispered.

"They buried the drawing with her and I went to the funeral and I cried so hard. I can remember thinking that I wanted to scale the exterior wall of the hospital and climb out onto the roof and shout to everyone in the world that Jessica was a beautiful girl, like a perfect snowflake sent from above, who had come to rest lightly in the palm of our hands. When she died, we were left holding only tears."

"There's so much sadness," I said.

"And so much happiness too," Brian answered. "There's no more beautiful reward than seeing a family come back to the hospital for a healthy, fun visit. There are a lot of children made well here, and when they stop by and say hello, or when they send a card to thank me, my God, it's wonderful. I must have an extended family of at least a hundred people, and I think of them so very often. I strive to be an example for others that work here, and let me tell you a secret." Brian leaned in for added affect. "My friend, I never worked with anyone here that I didn't genuinely like. Nor have I met a child who hasn't made me feel lucky, loved and filled with so many other emotions."

For me, it was too hard to comprehend. I thought about my own attitude and the moments when I didn't feel like being amiable to a co-worker, or a stranger who happened to get in my way. Certainly my own personality was worlds away from Brian's. "You must have had a wonderful childhood," I said.

Brian laughed heartily. "My God, no," he said. "I was born in Glasgow, Scotland. On January 2nd, 1953, I arrived at Ellis Island on the 2nd last voyage of Queen Mary."

"You're kidding, right?"

"No, my father was a man without a country and we were considered displaced people…refugees. My life as a child was messed up. We lived in a rundown, 18-story building in Astoria, Queens for three years before coming to Buffalo by train in 1956. I was only six years old but I remember that train ride as if it were this morning. That's one thing that I try not to forget; kids can remember. That's why I try to be happy for them when they're here. Someday, they'll remember being sick, and I want there to be some happiness in their memory banks."

Brian's eyes closed once more. He was traveling back through time to his own childhood. Unfortunately, what he was remembering was shrouded in a degree of pain. "In the early years we lived in Catholic Charity housing. The day after we arrived, there was a double homicide in our building. By the time I was eleven I had found a couple of dead bodies and witnessed two murders. We were dirt poor, brother. I remember having head lice, swatting roaches and wearing a rope on my pants to hold them up. When I was eight years old, I built my own shoeshine box, and I'd walk alone, for miles, to earn a buck or two. At ten, I was bailing newspapers in a junkyard. At twelve, I worked in a soda plant. Somehow I knew that keeping busy was the right thing to do."

I couldn't even imagine such an existence, let alone rising above it. Brian wasn't looking for my sympathy.

"Remembering the dark side of life makes you really want to do things that make others feel good. I truly believe that the negative things in life make you stronger and more acutely aware of the positive."

"It could've turned out differently," I said. "The streets are filled with people who don't make it out of difficult situations."

Brian sipped his soda and thought about it for a long moment. "You know, I could've taken the other road. I could've stayed pissed off forever, but I thank God that I didn't."

"And now here you are," I said, "experiencing every aspect of the human condition."

"Exactly," Brian answered, "and let me tell you, I'm open to everything. There are mornings when I get out of bed not knowing if it will be the happiest or saddest day of my life. I'll tell you something else; being here has allowed me to experience all cultures and races. I learned from the doctors and nurses that all personal beliefs have to be checked at the door. We all seem ready to work together to find a successful resolution. My friend, the only time I look down at someone is when I'm trying to help them up."

Brian shifted in his seat. At his right hand was a small hand-written note that was close enough to his computer monitor for him to see at all times. *"Dear Brian, Thank you so much for the check. It will help out with the cost of the guinea pig—as always your princess, Jessie.*

"There are days when the children need someone to be there. I'm lucky to be here. I'm unbelievably fortunate to be the guy that they ask to come into their life. So, you see, I have to be happy."

I asked Brian about his own children.

"Cameron is twenty now and Kari is twenty-four. They're both doing well and I'm just so grateful that they're healthy. They're wonderful children, I mean adults now, and I think about them when I'm hurting. I see myself in them, and that makes me more proud than I ever thought possible."

"Do you understand that your philosophy of life isn't shared by everyone?"

"Listen, I survived my childhood. I nearly drowned, survived typhoid fever, DDT poisoning and Legionnaires Disease. I have severe migraine headaches that just tear me up, but I never miss a day of work. Life is a miracle. Whether I meet you in the halls of the hospital or out on the street, I want you to remember me. I want to make a favorable impression. I want to send some happiness your way."

I extended my hand and Brian shook it quickly. "You've made a favorable impression on me."

"That's what it's all about, my brother," he replied with a smile.

I followed Brian back to the front of his office where the thank-you cards covered his walls. My eyes danced across a long, hand-written note from a child. I could only imagine the child as she worked to form each letter perfectly. At the bottom of the note was a tracing of the child's hand. Below the traced hands were the words: *"To Brian, I wanted you to have a picture of my patty. This is my patty."*

"Life is a miracle," Brian said. "We should let love give what it gives, without question, boundary, or reserve, for like life, love is a miracle too."

CHAPTER 7

The Story of Ellen Eckhardt, PICU Nurse

"Open your hearts to the love God instills…
God loves you tenderly.
What He gives you is not to be kept under lock and key,
but to be shared."
—Mother Teresa

There comes a time in everyone's life when they must chose a path to follow. Ellen Eckhardt decided her path at a very early age. "I always wanted to be a nurse," Ellen said as she sat down across from me in the hospital cafeteria. "My mother, Thelma, was a nurse and she's always been my favorite person in the world. I always wanted to be just like her." Ellen's eyes instantly filled with tears. I was surprised by the instantaneous show of emotion, and it occurred to me that perhaps we should have shifted the meeting as Ellen had just completed a twelve-hour shift. Ellen wiped away the tears and smiled. Her brown eyes sparkled, and it amazed me that she could pull it all together so quickly. She flicked her dark hair away from her face and clasped her hands on the table in front of her. "I'm just really surprised and grateful you'd want to talk to me about my job. This is like my second home. There are so many great things happening at the hospital now, and I'm grateful. This is where I love to be."

I allowed Ellen a moment to relax.

It was Ellen's soft, soothing approach to the job that appealed to my senses when my own son was in the need of care. Ellen had been Jake's nurse for quite a few days, and her professionalism was appreciated more than she'd ever know. Almost as if she were reading my mind, she verbalized the compassion that I'd long admired. "How's Jake?" she asked, "and your wife, Kathy, how is she? Is everyone well?"

"Jake is perfect," I said, "and Kathy and I are having a great time with all three of the boys."

"That's great. That's exactly what this job is all about. When a family leaves the unit, happy and healthy, it motivates me to do my job well. I always wanted to be a nurse because I've always had a real passion for people."

"You would have to in a job like yours," I said.

"There was a time," Ellen said, "when I remember wanting to go to Africa to tag animals. I always loved animals. In fact, my sister Diane and I used to mix dry milk with water every night, toss in the dinner scraps and head out to the barn to feed the animals. We used to do it every day, and I still have dreams that I forgot to feed the animals. Diane and I would stay out in the barn for hours taking care of the rabbits, cows, and sheep. I thought that I might work with animals, but Dad convinced me that nursing is more practical, so here I am. In fact, I owe a debt of gratitude to my father, Lester. He really led by example, and his work ethic always inspired me to do my best each day. I watched and worked with him on the farm, and his dedication to his work was incredible."

"Do you think your work taking care of the animals helped you decide to become a nurse?"

"I guess on some level. I always wanted to be a nurse, but I do remember when I was about eight my neighbor Larry fell out of a tree and was bleeding pretty badly. I was so upset at the sight of him being injured, but Larry recovered, and in seeing his injury and his healing something clicked."

Ellen explained she had graduated from Valparaiso University in 1983 with a bachelor of science degree in Nursing. "I've been here since June 21, 1983. I'm not sure how many people stay at their very first job, but it honestly is the team effort and the true professionals that surround me and keep me here."

"Have you always been in the Pediatric Intensive Care Unit?" I asked.

"I spent the first five years of my career in Variety 8, which is the surgical/orthopedic department, but I've been in the PICU ever since. When I started in the PICU, I was really quite over-whelmed, but Jennifer Josker, who was the Assistant Nurse Manager at the time, helped me do what I didn't think I could. Jennifer was able to guide and challenge me in such a way that I eventually gained confidence. Her belief in me has made a tremendous difference in my life."

I didn't want to sway the interview in any way, but I was a lit-tle biased. When Jake was at the hospital, the work of the nurses in the intensive care unit was simply fantastic. It didn't take long to answer the question of why the unit seemed to operate at such a high level.

"The team effort in the unit is unbelievable," Ellen said. "Each discipline of health care is extremely significant and every-one has a job to do. We respect each other, first and foremost, and it builds from there." Ellen leaned forward in her chair. "Each of our unit secretaries and administrative assistants are simply bom-barded with calls and visitors and all sorts of other distractions. They handle it very efficiently, which allows us to be at the bed-side, which is where we should be."

As Ellen spoke fondly of her co-workers, my mind drifted to an article that I'd read about the high stress of being a healthcare professional in a critical care unit. There was tremendous pres-sure steeped in the nature of the work. One simple mistake could potentially cause serious injury to the patient. Additionally, the article stated that many of the nursing units were short-staffed, putting extra pressure on each nurse. The hours were long, and the work could be grueling. Yet more than anything else, Ellen and the rest of the remarkable staff of nurses who made up the unit were forced, as an aspect of their job, to watch children suffer. The nurse was always at the very front line of human need and was expected to be strong in the face of family grief.

"There are so many ups and downs," Ellen said. "It's a challenging and rewarding job, and I don't know where I'd be if I wasn't here. I truly believe that God has a purpose for each and every one of us, and He carries it out in a grand design."

"You were born to be a nurse," I said again.

"No, actually, it's more than that," Ellen said. "It's more like there's a grand design for the sick child. We all have a role to play—the parents, the doctors, and the nurses. There are days when I wonder how I can possibly summon the strength to go into work. I pray for God to work through me. That's how I get through the difficult times. I learned early on in my career that you have to learn to separate real life from what's happening in the unit, but it's difficult to do."

The cafeteria was an extremely busy place. Over Ellen's shoulder I saw a group of nurses gathered at a table, sipping coffee and speaking in hushed tones. I simply couldn't imagine putting myself in a life or death situation each day. "What's the most difficult part of the job?" I asked.

"Watching a child suffer and not being able to make him or her well again," Ellen said. "It's also very difficult to see the parents suffering. When a child is sick, we get to see the parents when they're most vulnerable. Sometimes, we have to learn to deal with the anger, fear and devastation of the parents. In those cases, I so badly want to make the circumstances different, but I just can't. I've had cases where the parents have been angry or short with me, and I can't even tell you how much that hurts. I get through it by understanding there's no right or wrong way to grieve. Some people grieve by blaming someone else for their predicament, and as a nurse, I'm a convenient target sometimes. I understand that."

"Your coping skills must be phenomenal. Two questions here: How do you get through the stages of grief? And why do you put yourself through it?"

Ellen smiled. "I like to write," she said. "Ever since I was young, I've written down my thoughts as a way to work through them. Also, I pray a lot. I think that in my profession there has to be an ability to see the bigger picture. We all look at life a little differently, but there has to be something there for us to hold onto, you know?"

I nodded. There was little question that those in the health-care community leaned heavily on faith in God to get through the day. I considered that Ellen had referenced Psalm 46. She explained that it was a prayer she shared with her own children on an everyday basis.

> *God is our refuge and strength,*
> *an ever-present help in trouble.*
> *Therefore we will not fear,*
> *though the earth give way—*
> *And the mountains fall into the heart of the sea,*
> *Though its waters roar and foam and the mountains*
> *quake with their surging.*
> *There is a river whose streams make glad the city of God,*
> *The holy place where the Most High dwells.*
> *God is within her, she will not fall;*
> *God will help her at break of day.*
> *Nations are in uproar, kingdoms fall;*
> *he lifts his voice, the earth melts.*
> *The Lord Almighty is with us;*
> *the God of Jacob is our fortress.*
> *Come and see the works of the LORD,*
> *the desolations he has brought on the earth.*
> *He makes wars cease to the ends of the earth;*
> *he breaks the bow and shatters the spear,*
> *He burns the shields with fire.*
> *"Be still and know that I am God;*
> *I will be exalted among the nations,*
> *I will be exalted in the earth."*
> *The LORD almighty is with us;*
> *the God of Jacob is our fortress.*

"Why do I do it?" Ellen asked. "You know, I think about something a physician, David Steinhorn, told me a long time ago. He said, 'Ellen, it's not really about the child, it's about everyone taking care of the child.' I've found so much comfort in that because I understand my job is to make everything as comfortable as possible for that child." Ellen paused for a long moment. "It's difficult to explain, because, although it *is* about each and every child, it's also about how we come together as a team to make a difference for the child. It's almost as though everything slows down and I can see the subtle nuances of our interaction. I feel God gives us each a separate challenge in the care of that child. Do you know what I mean?"

I nodded, but I understood that Ellen was allowing me into a life that was more than I was prepared to comprehend.

"When I feel that all I can do isn't enough, I think of God and His challenge to me. It gives me the strength to make it through. It's not really about the child, it's about everyone taking care of the child."

"You mentioned writing," I said. "That's a subject near and dear to my heart. Tell me about how that helps you cope."

"A few years ago, after the loss of a patient, I sat at my kitchen table and I prayed. I was asking God why when it started to snow. It was like the first snowfall of the year when the flakes are really huge and form a blanket on the ground. I wrote a short story about a child asking her mother questions about life and how her mother's answers were meant to comfort her. I called it *Heaven's Blanket*. It comforted me to write it."

"Do you realize that you were meant to be a nurse?" I asked. "Think of it, it's a mother and a child and all of the hard questions of life. As a writer, you incorporated your strong faith and the thought that heaven wraps the child in a warm blanket. You have to share your story," I said.

"We'll see," Ellen said.

We were at the crucial stage of the interview. I had my question ready and I was certain that Ellen was waiting for it. There was no easy way to bring up the death of a child, but it was an aspect of the job that could not be avoided. Even though I was sure that my question would test the boundaries of Ellen's special heart, I forged ahead. "How does the unit cope with the loss of a child?"

The tears in Ellen's eyes betrayed the bravery shown in the rest of her interview. I was becoming proficient at recognizing the difference in the makeup of healthcare professionals as opposed to the rest of us.

"Each and every child is special," Ellen began. "Even if I never get the chance to meet them, I am exposed to the love. I see the love of the parents and the family. I see the love and it breaks my heart. I realize that I will never have the capacity to understand why a child dies, but I also see death as simply a stage of life. Death isn't final. My faith teaches me that death isn't final at all."

Ellen's voice faded. The rest of the cafeteria seemed to disappear from my view. I could only concentrate on her words and the unique make-up of the woman sitting across from me.

Ellen's eyes drifted away as she recalled a day long since past. "I often think of a darling little boy, Michael. He was so beautiful." Ellen's voice cracked with emotion and she deftly flicked a tear away. "He used to call me Dylan because he couldn't pronounce Ellen correctly." Ellen laughed and her eyes sparkled through the tears. "There are just so many moments in this job when you feel as though you're swinging from a pendulum. Michael was very sick, but there was a day when he was well enough to sit in a wheelchair. I took him out of the unit and we came down here to the cafeteria for a drink. Then he was able to sit out on the patio on the third floor with his parents. I stepped inside to give them some private time, but I was still able to see them. They talked of how the clouds made pictures in the perfect, blue sky. I can remember how bright the sun was shining and how happy I felt that he could feel fresh air. Michael's parents were just so grateful for that day." Ellen bowed her head. "Michael passed away a couple of days later. God gave Michael and his family that last beautiful moment."

Ellen's voice threatened to give way as she continued. "I

don't know how I do this," she said. "It's too emotional, it's too involved, and it's too intense. Sometimes there's just too much. Yet, you still feel the love more than anything else. There was another night that clearly sticks in my memory. Around Christmas one year, a baby passed away, and his parents were holding him for the very last time. After a long while, with my heart in my throat, I stepped into the room. The mother asked me if I would like to hold the baby, and I said, 'I would love to.' I held that baby as his mother began humming "Silent Night". It was such a beautiful moment. I sang softly to the baby, knowing that he felt the love in some way. The grief is so intense, but so is the love. Am I making sense?"

"Perfectly. You were born to be a nurse," I whispered.

Ellen forced a laugh that chased away the tears.

"Tell me about your happy days," I said.

"Oh Cliff, there are so many," Ellen said. "I remember the day when your son was having his surgery. Everyone on the unit was so nervous for you and your family. We were all praying, and when Jake was in surgery, you could hear a pin drop in that unit, but when he came out and we heard that everything was going to be all right, we were all ecstatic."

The tables had been turned as my own heart threatened to explode. "That's not fair," I whispered.

"There are so many days like that," Ellen said. "We all want to do our very best for every child. It sounds clichéd, but we are all one big family." As if to illustrate the point, Ellen removed a couple of photos from her pocketbook. I immediately recognized the face of Barb Koukanis, the driving force behind the Family-Centered Care Program at the hospital.

"That's Karen Mace, Barb and I. We took our mothers out for lunch one day and I took a few photos. I carry them with me all the time to remember that we are people who care for one another and who work together as a family."

"Tell me about your own family," I said.

"My partner and I have four children," Ellen said. She spread out the photos of her beautiful children. Ellen showed me photos of Zach, Sabrina, Anna, and Cole, who range in age from five to fifteen. "You talk about inspiration!" Ellen said. "They're so wonderful. Yesterday before I left for work, I just watched them sitting at the table eating dinner. They were talking and laughing and just sharing. I thank God every day that they're healthy. You know, every night we say prayers together and sing the song, *Make Me a Servant*. I just love being with them. I love taking care of them.

"You know why?" I asked.

"Why?" Ellen said.

"Because you're a nurse."

Ellen smiled.

"Are you going to share your writing with me?"

"We'll see," Ellen said.

CHAPTER 8

The Story of Anthony Stinson
Part II

"Let your courage mount with difficulties.
There would be no will if there were no resistance."
—*N.Sri Ram,* Thoughts for Aspirants

The slow decline of Anthony Stinson was not readily apparent to his family or to the doctors who were treating him. In many respects, there wasn't anything anyone could do to foresee the steady decline, because to be completely honest about it, those involved had no idea what they were up against. In early 2002, Anthony's condition worsened right before the very eyes of his family. Trina Stinson worked hard to make life normal for her sons, but Anthony was in pain, and it broke his mother's heart. "He used to pull at his hands and feet and yell, 'Hurt Momma,'" Trina said. "Imagine how that feels. He was in pain and I had no idea how to help him."

Trina was able to click off details about Anthony's illness as though the events are catalogued in her mind. "In February, 2002 Anthony was hospitalized for dehydration. He was throwing up blood, and he was just too weak to walk. Although we had no way of knowing it, it was simply the beginning of the nightmare. Anthony was hospitalized in March for tremors in his hands. It was so scary to watch, but one morning he just started to shake and I didn't know what to do. Of course, they ran a number of tests. During that particular visit, Anthony had a CT-Scan, an MRI, and a spinal tap. Everything came back normal. There wasn't an explanation for what he was going through." Trina looked at her son in the bed as she spoke. With a quick glance to the chalkboard that hangs in her living room, she leaned over and administered care to her son. Her movements were swift and direct and she smiled back in my direction. "Excuse me for a moment," she whispered.

I had no idea what Trina was doing, but every single moment of her life was dictated by the schedule on her wall to keep her son comfortable. I thought of the words, "Living a life of quiet desperation," but I immediately realized that what Trina is living is a life of absolute courage.

"Where were we?" Trina asked as she tucked a blanket around her son. "In April of 2002, Anthony was dehydrated again. The hand tremors passed as quickly as they came, but this time it was his mouth that started to violently tremble and shake. His arms were shaking too, as was his tongue as it protruded from his mouth."

I tried hard *not* to imagine the scene. I couldn't even begin to realize what Trina was feeling at the time, but I stopped myself from interfering with her thought process. Trina was doing her best to tell the story of her son as though he were simply a patient rather than her own flesh and blood. I understood that she needed to tell the story in such a manner, or she would never be able to get the words out.

"Anthony had another MRI on the 18th of April. I'll never forget the day because he was just so hyper and so on edge. He was in a lot of pain too, and everyone at the hospital was so afraid for all of us. I know it wasn't the cause of anything, but it seems to me that they administered Benadryl in Anthony's IV and immediately he tossed his head back and started choking. He wasn't breathing. I was absolutely out of my mind. My mom, Nan, was with me. I can never thank her properly for being there beside me."

Trina's voice trailed off. For the very first time, I felt as though the telling of the story might be too difficult. Yet Trina took a deep breath, stole another glance at her son, and then smiled at me. "We were trying so hard to get him to go to sleep. All parents understand that feeling, right? But Anthony kept throwing his head back violently. They gave him a suppository, but he screamed his way through that process and it didn't provide any relief."

"That had to be the most helpless feeling in the world," I whispered.

"My Mom and I sang 'Take Me Out to the Ballgame' over and over. Finally, Anthony calmed down, but the worst night of my life was just starting."

Like any other family, the Stinsons were not prepared for the night of April 19, 2002. Trina and Tom Stinson were supposed to be celebrating their fifth wedding anniversary. "It's simply amazing that the chapters of our family life seem to be separated by that date. The five-year anniversary," Trina said. She bowed her head and stared at the carpet, as though the answer to all of this was written on the floor. "Nicholas was almost four when Anthony got sick, and he handled it like a trooper. People tend to forget that behind every sick child that has to spend time in the hospital, there are very often other children and spouses who are left at home. I didn't leave the hospital for the first two weeks of Anthony's hospitalization. I sat in a chair beside his bed, ate horribly, drank too much coffee and just tried to exist. I had a burning desire to be there every moment, but as the Child Life Specialists explained, it doesn't do any good to run yourself into the ground. I felt like I had to, you know?"

Very often a parent of a sick child does exactly such a thing. I had a point of reference as I had felt exactly the same way when my own child was sick. I wanted to take some of the pain away from Jake, and I had figured that the best way to do such a thing was to run myself ragged. Of course, it was absolutely counterproductive to my son's care, as it was to Trina's son.

"After living at the hospital for two weeks, I couldn't function anymore. Over the course of the next four months, Tom and I would alternate nights at the hospital so that Nicholas was with one parent or another. What absolutely killed me was I wasn't able to do all of the things that a mommy should do. I wasn't there for Nicholas on a daily basis. I relied on others to raise my healthy son, and I often think of the time I missed with Nicholas, but what could I do? Nicholas would visit Anthony at the hospital and we would watch movies and play games, but that's a lot to ask of a four-year-old."

Trina could hardly speak of the guilt, but deep in her heart, she realized that she did all that she could. In her mind, it was never enough. Her time with a healthy Anthony was way too short, and realizing she missed some of Nicholas' development was even more disconcerting.

"I wish you could have seen Anthony when he was up and around," she said to me. "He was an absolute wild child. Even with his legal blindness and total unbalance he could not be stopped. Before he was hospitalized, Anthony pushed his way deep into the middle of anything that Nicholas and I were doing. I remember one afternoon Nicholas and I were trying to setup a racetrack. Anthony bullied his way in between and just annihilated the track. I told him that his middle name should be changed to 'Trouble' and Nicholas laughed hard. He wanted me to legally change Anthony's name."

Trina is a young woman, but it is certainly evident that the remainder of her days will be controlled by thoughts of lost days. "Anthony was so accident prone and wild," she said softly. "Even before he was incapacitated, I needed to be near him all the time. I protected him from everything because I had a wild fear that he would be hurt. I spent so much time and energy protecting him and caring for him I lost time just being a mom to my boys. I can't even begin to explain how that makes me feel."

Trina's self-doubt is certainly misplaced, but she is inconsolable on the issue. "Certainly, things could have been a lot different, but day-by-day you do what you think is right and after a while you wake up and realize your life has drastically changed."

The Stinsons never fully celebrated their five-year wedding anniversary. Beginning with the hospitalization of Anthony, the couple did their best to cope with the crippling force exerted on their marriage. "Tom did everything he could to work through the early months of Anthony's hospitalization. He took all of his vacation time, family leave time, and sick time, but eventually he had to go back to work. Unfortunately, life doesn't just stop because your child is sick. We needed to earn a living."

Nearly five years later, the Stinson marriage has dissolved. "There's so much there," Trina said, "but people need to know that when a child is as sick as Anthony is, sometimes the end of the marriage is a natural step. I don't know why it happens, and the particulars of our separation aren't as important as knowing it happens to couples on a regular basis. I go back to that night—April 19, 2002—and I understand that it was both the beginning of the end, and the start of a whole new life."

Trina was finally ready to talk about that night. "I don't know how many times my mother and I sang "Take Me Out to the Ball Game". Anthony finally fell asleep, but he kept waking up and he was just so uncomfortable. He alternated between choking on his own secretions and being totally unresponsive. The ICU fellow ordered Atavan, but that didn't help. At one o'clock in the morning I called Tom and asked him to bring a CD player and the Shania Twain CD." Trina smiled at the thought of using the CD as a sedative for her critically ill son. "I used to sing and dance with the boys as we listened to the CD. We calmed Anthony with our singing, so I figured that perhaps more music would help. I guess what it comes down to is that I also understood that Anthony was in serious trouble and I thought that Tom needed to be there."

Trina's mind is devoid of the details of the next five hours. "I spent a lot of time staring into space. Anthony was on the 7th floor. I spent most of the time just moving back and forth in a rocking chair. What is the proper response when your child is choking on his own secretions and is completely unresponsive? I guess I'll never know."

In the living room of her home, with her sick son lying beside her, and her healthy son playing with small racecars with one ear on his mother's words, Trina continued. It is a story that she has told over and over, but the pain in her heart is evident as her words reach my ears. "At six in the morning, Anthony went into a prolonged seizure. They call it status epilepticus. The staff from the Intensive Care Unit met us on the 7th floor and quickly whisked Anthony to the ICU. The single image that haunts me, day after day, is seeing Anthony's tiny hand hanging over the side of the bed. His hand was shaking because of the seizure." Trina's voice dropped almost to a whisper. I couldn't tell if it was because Nicholas was listening, or due to strong emotion. "His tiny hand in seizure is burned into my memory. It breaks my heart to even say the words."

Trina stepped off the bed and immediately reinstalled the rails so that Anthony couldn't possibly roll out of the bed. It was plain to me to see that he will not be rolling, but Trina was quick and deliberate in her movements. She glanced up at the chalkboard, but quickly returned her attentions to me. "A PICU resident came into the waiting room and asked me so many questions about Anthony. As I spoke with him, I just sat on the floor of the waiting room with my arms wrapped around my knees. I did my best to answer his questions, but it felt like an out-of-body experience. It felt like a lifetime, but I'm sure that just a few hours passed before we were able to see Anthony. By this time, Anthony was in a medically-induced coma to eliminate the seizures, but we just weren't prepared for what we saw. This was our boy! Anthony had EEG leads wrapped in gauze around his head. He was intubated, which is when a tube is placed down his throat and stabilized with tape around his mouth. He was on a ventilator and was catherized. Anthony had an arterial line stitched into his wrist and a central line stitched into his groin. There were three other IVs that looked like they had a hundred ports to administer meds. My boy was hooked to a pulse ox monitor, a heart monitor and a respiration monitor. I didn't know what any of it meant, and sometimes when I close my eyes at night, I can see him there, buried underneath all of that equipment."

Trina's confusion on that night seems misplaced as I realized that she was now caring for Anthony with very limited assistance.

"It was really difficult to think or talk or even stand up straight. I couldn't understand much, but the nurses and doctors were simply wonderful. They were not only taking care of Anthony, but they were taking care of us too. I didn't fully appreciate their compassion on the first night, though, because it was just too much. I wasn't in any position to truly understand."

There was little doubt that Trina was in a state of shock on that first night.

"The next day was just as difficult to comprehend. Anthony was having break-through seizures, but I just couldn't even look at him. As the day wore on, I found that I could not physically walk into the room. I wanted to go in, and my brain was screaming at me to be by his side, but I couldn't make my feet move. Instead, I flopped down in the darkened waiting room. I wasn't even sitting on a piece of furniture. I must have made a hell of a sight, sitting in the room with my legs wrapped in my arms, staring off into space."

Trina's reaction was certainly in line with what was happening, but a PICU attending physician finally broke through the storm in her brain. He met with Trina in PICU room #3.

"Dr. Rotta spoke with us about what they thought had happened to Anthony. I'll never forget it because he spoke to me in such a soothing voice. Dr. Rotta explained that it was possible that Anthony had a mitochondrial disease called Leigh's Disease. Of course, I had no idea what he was speaking of, but he laid it all out for us in simple terms. He was so compassionate and so caring." Again, Trina's voice faded a bit. She walked around the room slowly, glanced at Anthony, and then turned to see if Nicholas was still listening to our discussion. Nicholas had retreated into another room where he was watching television, worlds away from that horrific day.

"I asked Dr. Rotta what could be done. I was looking for a bottom line answer. I wanted to know what the cure was and how quickly it could happen for us. Dr. Rotta wasn't in any position to tell me what I needed to hear. Instead, he explained that there wasn't a cure for the disease that Anthony might have. He explained to me that my son was going to degenerate over the next couple of years, and that he would eventually die."

Trina removed the rail from the bed and sat back down next to her son. She forced a smile that was simply a gesture made to contradict how she had felt at that very moment. "I fell on the floor," she said. "My legs just cut out and I landed right there in front of Dr. Rotta. I had no idea what to do to even stand up straight. I don't know how long I stayed there on the floor, but eventually Tom and I made it to the hospital chapel on the 4th floor. We cried and prayed for a long while. We took a walk outside to get some air, but nothing at all made sense to me. There was just a huge cloud of confusion surrounding us. Looking back on it, I just didn't have a coherent thought in my head."

Trina shook her head and a slight smiled returned. "It's impossible to try and gauge how much you can handle as a human being. What I learned most of all was that I had an enormous reservoir of strength. At the moment when I fell to the floor in his PICU room, I didn't think that there would ever be another normal second in my life. I had also underestimated the love that I felt for my son. When people wonder how I make it through the dark days of Anthony's illness, I have to smile because I know that there are no limits to my love."

As it turned out, the tests that were administered on that first day came back normal. Anthony, while following all the patterns, did not have Leigh's Disease. "Dr. Rotta apologized to me for scaring us, but we definitely understood. It's so difficult for the staff at the hospital. They don't want to bring bad news, but they have to explain everything, regardless of how devastating the news might be."

The true testament of Trina's strength, love, and compassion came ringing through when she spoke of the doctors, nurses, social workers, Child Life, and secretaries at The Women and Children's Hospital of Buffalo. "It's a wonderful place," Trina said. "Every single person that we met treated us as special human beings. I simply can't put it all into words. There we were, receiving the worst possible news, and we were grateful for the dedication of the staff and those involved with Anthony's care. They always made us feel comfortable. They listened to my fears. They helped me through the tears. Basically, they were there for me whenever I needed them to be. All of the doctors involved were true professionals. My heart swells when I think of the compassion of Dr. Furman, Dr. Joshi, Dr. Budi, Dr. King, Dr. Hernan, and Dr. Rotta, and the nurses! Oh My God, the nurses were just so supportive."

I knew what Trina was feeling as she ticked off the names of all of those who supported her in her time of need. I remembered feeling such an overwhelming sense of gratitude that it was impossible not to tear up. Trina's eyes threatened tears as she recited the names of those who helped her family. "Every single nurse helped me. I think of Deb Powers, Barb Kourkounis, Sheila, Peggy, Rich and Linda. They were Anthony's nurses in the ICU and there were so many more. I am not exaggerating when I say that they were all truly wonderful. On the 7th floor our nurses were Aimee Horan and Eileen English, but it's hard to be specific because every single one of them deserves my thanks."

Trina paused for a moment. It appeared that she was begging her mind to provide her with the names of the people that she needed to say thank-you to. "There was Merril, Kathy, Patty, Vicki, Lisa and Karen. I truly want the people of Western New York to know that this hospital is an unbelievable place. If it wasn't for the kindness, dedication and genuine caring shown to us by the staff, I'm not sure that I could have possibly coped with Anthony's illness."

In an effort to give Trina a break from recounting the story of discovering Anthony's illness, I leaned out of my chair and picked up a slip of paper on the side table. It was a single sheet of 8 x 11 paper that has the words *Anthony Stinson's Medications* type-written across the top. I glanced at the sheet, understanding that I didn't have the capacity to understand what had truly happened to the Stinson family.

The sheet read: **Clonazepam** (0.5 mg/pill)—1 pill at 2 a.m., 1 p.m., 8 p.m.—½ pill at 8 a.m./ **Phenobarb** (30 mg/pill)—1 pill at 3 a.m., ½ pill at 11 a.m., 1 pill at 7 a.m./ **Valproic Acid** (250 mg/5 ml)—5 ml at 5 a.m., 10 ml at 2 p.m., 10 ml at 9 p.m./ **Zantac** (15 mg/ml—75 mg/5ml) 2.5 ml at 7 a.m., 2.5 ml at 7 p.m./ **Pulmicort** (0.5/2 ml/respule) 1 respule at 11 a.m., 1 respule at 11 p.m./ **Vitamin E** (400 iu) 1 a.m./ **Polyvisol with Iron**—1 ml at 3 a.m./ **Folic Acid** (1 mg/tablet) 1 pill at 1 a.m./ **Hydrocortisone** (liquid cortef, 2 ml/1 ml)—give with 20 ml liquid yogurt STRESS DOSE: 5 ml tip X 2 days/ **Dilantin** (50 mg/chewable pill)—2 pills at 10 a.m./ 3 ½ pills at 11 p.m./ **Prilosec** (2 mg/ml) 20 ml liquid yogurt ½ later 10 ml via JT at 8 a.m./ **IVIG** (15 grams) 1 time per month/ **Carnitor** (Liquid give with 20 ml liquid yogurt) 5 ml at 5 a.m., 5 ml at 2 p.m., 2 ml at 9 p.m./ **Ascorbic Acid** (500 mg/5 ml syrup) 2.5 ml at 1 a.m./ **237 ml Kindercal** with fiber 573 ml **Kindercal**—continuous thru JT over 13.5 hours/ **Water**—800 ml over 24 hours/ **Lacto-bacillus** Granules lactinex—1 package in food/ **Levothyroxine** (.025 mg/pill) 1 ½ pill at 5 p.m.

I held the slip of paper in my hand reading the names of the medications over and over. When I looked up at Trina again, it was through eyes of utter amazement. Each and every day is consumed with Anthony's care, yet she has also found the time to raise Nicholas, attend parent advisory meetings at the hospital, and amazingly enough, still smile. "How can you possibly manage this?" I asked.

"Remember that unlimited love I was speaking of?" Trina answered. She turned to face Anthony. I realized the story was just beginning.

CHAPTER 9

The Story of Deborah King & Child Life Services

"Thank you, Lord,
for the sheer joy of wanting to get up
and help the world go around."
—*Roxie Gibson*

In the playroom of Variety-9 of the Women and Children's Hospital, a Buffalo Sabres autographed jersey of legendary hockey player Pat LaFontaine hangs on one wall. There are four X-Box game consoles, Nintendo game consoles, four computers and a plasma television set. In the corner bookcase are a number of board games that will help sick children pass the time. Sorry, Life, Clue, Monopoly, Chutes & Ladders and Candyland are all there, waiting for a child to open up the box. In surveying the room, one feels a sense of true accomplishment, since the staff, along with Mr. LaFontaine, and the giving people of Western New York, has banded together to assist children who find themselves in a difficult situation. There is also a sense of dread and despair that sweeps over any visitor to this room. Children should be allowed to play with their toys at home in the safe, secure presence of an innocent world.

"It's a privilege to work with sick children," Deborah King explained. The motto of the Child Life Department is "Child's Play is a Serious Matter". My family and friends think that it's depressing to work with sick children, but I must tell you, our work is uplifting. I'm very happy to be a part of the team."

Pat LaFontaine's vision of a playroom was fully realized, and the state-of-the-art room brought a tear of gratitude to the heart. "We have web cameras installed so that children from our hospital can communicate with children at other facilities. There is also a pod with a web camera that allows children to see their family. It's a wonderful room, but we aren't done growing, either. We are looking to redo the adolescent playroom on Variety-10. The plan is to turn the room into a movie theatre with a video arcade. Our departmental goal is to allow for a bit of normalcy in a truly abnormal setting."

Deborah King moved through the hospital with grace and ease. In her movements, it was easy to recognize that she is proud of the achievements of her staff and the work they do on a daily basis. As I shadowed her through the hallways on Variety-9, my eyes were drawn to the beautifully decorated walls with the caricatures of animals, sunsets and rainbows. I thought back in time to when Jake was in the hospital and I realized that what was flooding my heart was absolute gratitude. Jake and I had entered the playroom long before it had been redone. In a moment that will stay with me until the end of time, I had stood across from my very sick child and played a game of air hockey. The sounds of his laughter, on that day long since past, still rang in my ears.

"It sounds clichéd, but everyone on the staff treats each and every child as if they're their own. Who wouldn't want a job where you get to help as many people as you can?" Deborah asked.

Again, I thought of my own children as I scanned the playroom. Without question, my healthy children would welcome the idea of staying in the room and playing as the hours pass. "My kids would love it here," I said.

"We want all the kids to love it here," Deborah replied.

The Child Life Department at The Women & Children's Hospital of Buffalo is so much more than a playroom, however. "We have a definite purpose and some serious goals," Deborah explained. "It may seem like I come into work just to play, but all of my thoughts center around providing emotional support to the hospital patients and their families. Listen, there's a lot of anxiety associated with a hospital visit. Our department helps children to feel as comfortable as they can in their new surroundings."

Together we traveled from the playroom on Variety-9 to the Child Life Offices on the 2nd floor. Deborah's office was filled with boxes of children's books, DVDs and computer games. "We recently had a very sizable donation. If you're writing the story of Child Life, you must include something about the wonderful people of Western New York. Everyone is so generous, from the sports teams, to the business community, to the individual people who love this place. They make our jobs so much easier."

Deborah cleared space at a table just off the main offices of The Child Life Department. We sat across from one another, both realizing that we were there to speak about bringing a little sunshine to what is normally a dark experience.

"Parents don't want to bring their children to the hospital, and children don't want to be here. There's a lot of fear and anxiety involved. We greet the family and try to take away some of the stress. Plain and simple, our staff is here to help." Deborah paged through some notes she had gathered for the meeting. She smiled broadly as she extended a full-page photograph of a family dressed for an old-fashioned tea party. Along with staff members, the family played dress-up one afternoon with fancy hats, colorful beaded necklaces and wide smiles. On the table before them was a sterling silver teakettle and fancy-flowered cups. "This is a family that wanted to have an old English tea party. The staff gathered some items and we staged the event. We all laughed so hard."

I was awestruck by the smiling faces in the photograph. "I can't even tell who's sick," I said.

"That's the idea," Deborah answered.

"Everyone is just so happy."

"The corporate line on the Child Life Department is that we are here to provide support, facilitate coping, minimize emotional trauma, and encourage normal growth and development for infants, children and adolescents. I like to think that it's much simpler than that: We're here to make people happy."

I couldn't imagine that Deborah had anticipated such a life. After graduating from the University of Iowa with a bachelor of sciences degree in Psychology, Deborah settled in as a teacher of functional behavior.

"In Iowa the work I was doing was to teach children appropriate behaviors as opposed to negative behavior responses. There wasn't the emotional connection to the children as there is here at The Women & Children's Hospital. Here, I'm just as likely to end up at a tea party as I am in assessing behavior."

"Tell me about your staff," I said.

"My God, it's a wonderful department," Deborah said. "On staff we have Dena Stearns, Tara Young, and Maureen McOwen. We also have a Child Life Specialist in training, McKenzie Mattison. The reason why I say it is such a wonderful staff is because we all enjoy what we're doing."

"All right, let's get into it," I said. "Tell me how it works."

"One of our most important functions is to assist a child in the preparation for surgery. If your child is here for surgery, we'll meet with him or her and show videos or use pictures to explain the procedure. We'll talk very softly and use a million corny jokes to take the stress out of the situation. In a lot of cases, we'll use dolls to show the child how the doctors and nurses might handle the procedure. We'll let them touch the medical equipment and even use it on us. We turn the tables a little so that when they are actually preparing for the surgery, they've already been through a dress rehearsal."

"So, what it does is allow the child to feel comfortable," I said.

"We're in the business of taking away the shock and the awe. You know, it's funny, but sometimes the parent needs Child Life Services more than the child. We are provided detailed information that allows us to comfort both mother and child."

"Or father and child," I said. My mind drifted back to Jake's hospital stay. During one of the first three days we were in the

PICU, Maureen McOwen had paid a visit to my son. Maureen's presence was like a true beacon of light during an extremely stressful time. She had offered Jake movies, cartoons, and even a small blue bank to take his mind off the tests and needle sticks. I shared the story with Deborah and she smiled. "We've touched a lot of lives," she said. "How can it possibly be anything but rewarding?"

"You must love children," I said in what must have been the understatement of the year.

"I've always been a kid magnet," Deborah answered, "but what really changed things for me was having my own children. Nathan was born in 2002, and Peter came two years later. Everyone says having children will cause your priorities to change, but it's even more pronounced when you are coming into this environment on a daily basis. It's impossible not to thank your lucky stars every day when you see how many truly sick children there are."

"Here's the million-dollar question," I said.

Deborah leaned forward in the chair. "How do I handle seeing one sick child after another?"

"Exactly," I said.

"Insomnia," Deborah answered with a laugh. "It's impossible not to let it affect you personally, but in my heart I know we are trying to help as many children as we can. The thought gets all of us through the day."

Deborah paused for a moment and I immediately recognized she was doing something that each and every staff member of the hospital was prone to do. Rather than accepting my amazement at her individual effort, she was comfortable speaking of others.

"The doctors and the nurses simply amaze me," she said. "The staff will contact us to meet with children. I am amazed with the abilities of the doctors and even more amazed with their sense of true compassion. There are a lot of people here who see the parade of sick children, and still perform. The Child Life staff understands that we have a place in the care of the children, and we realize that we are important."

Deborah paged through her notes again. She slipped a pamphlet across the table to me. "On Saturday mornings at 11 a.m. we offer orientations for children who are scheduled to come into the hospital for a procedure. One member of the staff will give a tour to the children. We teach them how to put on masks, we show them the game room, let them look through our collection of DVDs and books. Most every Saturday, we leave them clapping and smiling as they get ready for their stay with us. It's an opportunity for the parents and the children to become acquainted with the sights, sounds, smells, places and people of the hospital in a more relaxed atmosphere."

Above all else, it was easy to recognize that Deborah was passionate about the hospital and the care that each child receives. "Both of my sons have had to visit the hospital as patients," Deborah said. "As a parent, you're out of your mind with worry, and as a child you're unbelievably apprehensive about coming here. I am living proof of the job that our department does. My visit here as a patient was comfortable because of the staff of people that helped us cope."

"We have a number of other services that you probably don't even know about," Deborah said. "We have a program called *Helping Children Grow Through Grief* that is a bereavement support group for children from five to sixteen years of age."

Deborah handed me a pamphlet that I glanced at as she spoke. My eyes darted to a quotation in the center of the first page: *"Some people come into our lives, leave footprints on our hearts, and we are never the same."*

"The children's support group focuses on providing age-appropriate activities for expression of some common emotions felt after loss," Deborah explained. "We give children an opportunity to voice memories."

The *Helping Children Grow Through Grief* group meetings are held on the second Wednesday of every month at the First Trinity Lutheran Church in Tonawanda, New York.

Deborah had one more slip of paper in her hand. She slid it across the desk to me and I glanced down at *Relaxation Techniques*.

"Parents and patients alike often are in a state of shock when they come through the doors for the first time. As the pamphlet explains, you'll never know what might relax you. Every single person reacts to stress in a different manner. We try to make it easier for the patient by explaining some of the more common relaxation techniques."

The pamphlet explained breathing exercises, guided imagery techniques, attention diversion techniques, progressive muscle relaxation, and meditation techniques.

"I could have used this when we were here," I said. "I kind of missed what everyone was saying to me at that time."

"That happens too."

Deborah leaned back in her chair and smiled. "I keep saying it, but we are here to help."

"What's the best part of your job?" I asked.

"The team concept of healthcare at the hospital is terrific. I love the people that I work with on a daily basis, and we all have the same goal—to make the children comfortable. Yet, there are so many fun times. We celebrate the holidays with the children. We're here to cheer on the Sabres and the Bills. We even had SabreTooth, the team mascot, in here to visit the children, and the ward just came alive. The players visit from time-to-time too, and everyone gets so excited."

Deborah's eyes danced with excitement when she was simply talking about the children. "If we can reduce some of the trauma, and if a child remembers us, it is all so worthwhile. We have families return to say hello, and I can't tell you how good it feels to see a happy, healthy family. There's nothing better than that."

"And yet, some children don't get to go home," I said.

"It's like the movie *Pollyanna*," Deborah said. "Sometimes I walk around wondering, what's good about this? Still, we try and help make it as normal as we can. There are children who come to us that have just a limited amount of time left. We owe it to the family and parents to cry with them. When a patient dies, it is sad for all of us, there's no getting around that. I try not to be too emotional, but it's hard. When it happens, I feel like a daughter to some of the parents and a friend to others. I've gone to the funerals of patients who've passed away, and I've had parents consoling me!"

Deborah's demeanor was free and easy. She had long ago accepted the difficult part of her job. It is a job that not a lot of people could do, but she has made her peace with all of it. "I feel that it's part of my job to honor the spirit of that child. I am honored that I have had the chance to work with them."

Deborah led me through the back offices of the Child Life Department. We stopped long enough to say hello to McKenzie Mattison, a Child Life specialist in training. Deborah waved her hand around the room as if to show me the spirit and the generosity of the Western New York Community. There are books, games, and DVDs stacked as high as the eye can see. "We can't even begin to thank everyone who donates to us. You asked me what the reward is, and its always right in front of me. I see the good things every single day. It would be easy to get down about the sickness. No child should ever have to go through some of the things that these kids go through, but it would be wrong to be sad about it. The Child Life Department exists to help. Let everyone know that we are excited to have the chance to work with sick children and their families."

CHAPTER 10

The Story of Dr. Michael Caty
Part I

"This is the true joy in life,
the being used for a purpose recognized by yourself
as a mighty one;
the being thoroughly worn out before you are
thrown on the scrap heap;
the being a force of nature instead of a feverish selfish
little clod of ailments and grievances
complaining that the world will not devote itself
to making you happy."
—*George Bernard Shaw*

I will truly never forget the moment when I met Dr. Michael Caty. The date was November 5, 2001, on the 2nd floor of The Women and Children's Hospital of Buffalo. Dr. Caty entered the surgical waiting room at a little after noon with the purpose of explaining to my family how the surgery had gone on my son Jacob. When I close my eyes and concentrate, I can clearly see the complex look on Dr. Caty's face that day. The look in his eyes was one of relief, compassion, and satisfaction. He wiped his tired brow and smiled at us. "The surgery went very well," he said. He led us to a table in the conference room just off the waiting room. In the simplest of terms he explained what the team had accomplished. Dr. Caty concluded the discussion by saying that, after a short recovery, Jake would be returning home with us as good as new. He spoke the words, with tears of relief in his eyes. At that moment, I saw everything I needed to know about the man. He was driven in his work; proud of the accomplishments of the hospital; and ultimately immersed in the business of helping children.

On that day, I hugged my wife, my mother, my father, my sister, my brother, and sister-in-law. I also hugged Dr. Caty as if he were a member of my family. Five years later, as I write these words, I can clearly say, without reservation, that Dr. Caty is a welcome member of a great number of families across Western New York. Yet there is so much more to this remarkable man, that it would be a shame to write a story of the hospital and not include his life's story.

The biographical information of Michael Caty is truly impressive, but words on paper do little to describe his dedication and commitment to The Women & Children's Hospital of Buffalo, and the Western New York Community. Dr. Michael Caty lives his life with a true sense of purpose and dedication.

I had long looked forward to spending time with Dr. Caty. My goal in the interview was to capture the true spirit of the man. Rather than simply listing his accomplishments, I wanted to talk with Dr. Caty and show that he is a deeply introspective man who carries each and every one of his patients in his heart. I was certain that the two hours I would spend with him would change me in some fashion.

I entered Dr. Caty's office on a bright, sunny morning in September of 2006. At precisely 10:00, Dr. Caty entered the reception area and extended his hand to me. "So good to see you," Dr. Caty began. It was a typical greeting, but Dr. Caty's tired eyes came alive when he said the words, and I knew that he meant it. I was used to the greeting, however, because it was something that he'd said to me each time in the past five years, and it always made me feel accepted. I followed Dr. Caty into his office and sat in a chair across from him. He was dressed in green surgical clothes, and he looked drawn, as though he'd been up all night.

"Thank you for taking the time to speak with me," I said.

"It's good for the hospital," Dr. Caty answered. "I'm always willing to do my part."

"That's a good way to start," I said. "I've spoken with a number of people on staff here at the hospital, and I'm impressed with the team concept that everyone preaches. I'm beginning to understand the workings of a top-notch women and children's hospital."

Dr. Caty smiled. He has a bright, infectious smile that he makes good use of as he speaks to his patient's families. "We have a group of individuals here who are the core fiber of what we do. People working together on a common goal are what makes for a successful hospital."

"I must tell you that in the interview process many of the staff comment about *your* demeanor. From the nurses to the chaplain to the Child Life Department, everyone comments about how comfortable you make them feel as you go about your work."

"I appreciate that," Dr. Caty said. "I think it's important to talk and listen to the people you work with on a daily basis. I am on a first-name basis with all of the staff, including the grounds-keepers, the housekeepers and the nursing staff. I think it's important to work that way because everyone has something to offer. For instance, I had a conversation in passing one morning with a groundskeeper. Jim mentioned to me that it would be better for our patients if there were a covered bus stop that would provide shelter in bad weather. It was an exceptional idea, and now we have a covered bus stop. Jim's ability to see things made a difference around here, and I'm a believer in working together. We're all in this to make the hospital a better place, and that's how things work sometimes."

"That's understood," I said. "But there are long hours and a lot of difficult cases. It must be difficult to stay upbeat all the time."

"Not really," Dr. Caty answered. "A long time ago, back in medical school, I tried hard to recognize and adopt the best trait from each individual I would meet. I still try and live that way.

Besides, I'm conditioned to be upbeat. In my job, I strive to be a source of hope, and it works much better if I stay positive."

"Which brings me straight to the heart of the matter," I said. "It's a question that I've brought up in each interview for this story. How do you handle the endless parade of sick children?"

"It's what all of us aspire to do," Dr. Caty said. "We have a job to do and we must maintain high standards. It's all about professionalism. As surgeons, we take an oath of professionalism, and as surgeons, there really isn't anyone watching us when we're performing surgery. There may be a moment when we ask ourselves if we really need to put the extra stitch in. We owe it to ourselves and our patients to maintain professionalism, and we put the extra stitch in."

"Yet, given your high level of performance and the number of years you've been doing this work, there must be a temptation to say, 'I've seen my share of sick children.' You're a successful man."

"I believe that if you work hard, success will come to you. Yet, more than anything else, men and women enter this profession to help people, and that's at the center of it all."

Dr. Caty moved to his desk and quickly retrieved three slips of paper. He extended them to me in an effort to explain his motivations. On the first slip of paper were quotations from Theodore Roosevelt and George Bernard Shaw. The second sheet contained the words of the Oath of Maimonides. "The motivation to do well is contained in the words of the oath I took."

Oath of Maimonides

"Thy eternal providence has appointed me to watch
Over the life and health of my fellow human beings.
May the love for my art actuate me at all times;
May neither avarice nor miserliness, nor thirst for
Glory, or for great reputation engage my mind; for
The enemies of truth and philanthropy could easily
Deceive me and make me forgetful of my lofty aim
Of doing good to my patients. May I never see in

The patient anything but a fellow creature of pain.
Grant me strength, time, and opportunity,
Always to correct what I have acquired,
Always to extend its domain; for knowledge is immense
And the spirit of man can extend infinitely
To enrich itself daily with new requirements.
Today we can discover our errors of yesterday
And tomorrow we may obtain a new light on what
We think of ourselves sure of today.
I have been appointed to watch over the life and
Death of my fellow human beings. Here am I ready
For my vocation and now I turn unto my calling."

The third slip of paper contained an underlined passage of words that fully explained Dr. Caty's motivations. The quotation was contained in the preface to the Pediatric Life Support Book. *Yet those of us who take care of children know better. We know that children are a rejuvenating wellspring of love and wonder, and caring for them nurtures us as well as them. We know that our work results in more laughter, more discovery, more sleepovers, more birthday parties, more cupcakes, more dances, more graduations, and eventually more of us. It is my belief that nowhere are the stakes higher or the rewards greater than in the care of critically ill children. It is our duty and our privilege to do our best. Those of us who have dedicated our lives to caring for ill children have done so because we understand these things.*

As I read the words, my heart swelled because I was sitting directly across from a man who had helped to grant my own child more days of happiness and discovery. I certainly could understand how unbelievably satisfying the profession could be. Still, there were pitfalls that needed to be discussed.

"I recently read an article that explained that despite the success of their professional lives, a great number of surgeons commit suicide," I said. "That surprised me."

"There's a great need for balance in our lives," Dr. Caty explained. "Some surgeons run the risk of having their lives slip out of balance. Let's face it, the hours are long, the work is difficult, and there is a great deal of responsibility. It is oftentimes very difficult to balance our professional lives and our personal lives."

"Tell me about a typical day," I said.

Dr. Caty smiled. His tired eyes flashed a cynical look as though I would not be able to fully digest what he would consider a typical workday. He was absolutely correct in his assumption.

"Last night I finished up here at around ten o'clock. I had a late dinner with my wife, got some rest, and was up at 5 a.m. to take my son to crew practice. I was here before six this morning and I'll do whatever needs to be done through the day. In this profession there are high rates of divorce, alcoholism, and suicide, but you owe it to everyone you work with to find the balance. It's difficult sometimes, but I find the time to spend with my family, and to exercise, and live a little. It's dependent upon choices that we make. I wouldn't consider my life as being successful had I shortchanged my family in some way."

Dr. Caty had been correct: I couldn't fathom such a schedule on a routine basis. I shook my head in amazement and he quickly caught on to my sense of disbelief.

"As doctors we are conditioned to those types of hours. As you work your way through medical school and through the residency program, everything else takes a back seat. During residency, we are expected to be on duty every other night through the night. The typical schedule has you reporting to work on say, Monday morning, and you work through the entire day and all of the next day. For five to seven years, we are asked to stay awake through the night, every other night. It is not easy to condition yourself to do such a thing, but it's part of the discipline."

"And you've been able to maintain a balance?"

"I've always enjoyed outside reading, and sports too, but there are choices to make. I don't golf because, although I might like to, I can't take such a huge block of time away from my family. It isn't fair to them. I also enjoy sailing, but once again, the time commitment is too much. So, there are days when I have to exercise at 5 a.m. It's part of the job."

I knew for certain that my mind was not quite strong enough to handle such a schedule, but Dr. Caty went out of his way to make sure that I understood where he was coming from.

"I consider myself incredibly fortunate to be in this position," he said. "I have a magnificent job where I have the opportunity to make children healthy. So, I work thirteen or fourteen hours a day; it's part of the responsibility."

"Do you ever feel rested?" I asked.

Dr. Caty hesitated for a long moment and then smiled. "Not really," he said with a chuckle. "Right at the tail end of my vacation I'll feel nearly rested, but then I return to work."

What entered my mind at that moment were the expectations of a family as they meet a surgeon for the first time. Most people had very little understanding of the unselfish nature of the job and the sacrifice made on a daily basis. As patients, we expected our surgeons to be perfect, against all odds, and in the face of some of life's greatest challenges. Unfortunately, when the outcome isn't exactly what was expected, we hold those surgeons responsible.

"I know I'm going to get your dander up a bit, but it's pretty easy to sue a doctor in this day and age."

Dr. Caty shifted in his seat. For the very first time, his expression changed as his smile dimmed. "I can honestly say that I have always been well-prepared for surgery. My goal is to do my job to the best of my ability, but surgery is an imperfect world." Dr. Caty chose his words carefully because it was most certainly a subject that was difficult to address. "I had a process server show up at my house and tell one of my children that I was being sued. It's not an easy situation to confront. Listen, we aren't in there doing stupid things. There are simply no guarantees. I begin each operation or case with the idea that this is how I would proceed if this were my child who needed help."

"It's too bad that in this day and age people need to find somewhere to put the blame," I said.

"As surgeons, we are extremely possessive and obsessive. It's very easy to forget about all of our successes and dwell on our failures. It's another trap of the profession, but as caring individuals, we are more concerned about what could have been done differently. I've lost a lot of sleep over that through the years, but yes, I wish the system of blame were approached differently. We continue to address those types of situations here also. Once a month, we meet as a team to discuss difficult cases and complications. We meet in an effort to eliminate potential mistakes."

"You mentioned that, as a surgeon, you are obsessive and possessive with your work. I imagine that those traits would be difficult to turn off around the home."

"Not really," Dr. Caty said. His smile returned as he addressed his true passion: his own family. "There isn't anyone handing me things at home," he said. "The person I am at work couldn't truly function in the home environment. I can't direct the people I love as I might have to in a work setting. It's all part of that balance."

"Yet it must be difficult to check your emotions at the door."

"Certainly, but my wife, Diana, is a wonderful, supportive, strong, independent person. There is such a high volume of emotional content that just can't spill over at home. Diana is extremely supportive, but it wouldn't be fair of me to burden her with all of the specific information of my hospital life. Diana's family was heavily involved in medicine, so she understood the life of a surgeon. Her grandfather and father were surgeons and her four siblings are physicians."

"Diana is also an attorney," I said.

"Yes, and a strong, independent woman, and I am blessed to be married to her. In a surgeon's life, there are all sorts of sacrifices involved. Through the years, Diana had to do a lot of the heavy lifting around the house. I was certainly there to discipline the children and love the children, but she handled most of the day-to-day responsibility. When you talk about balancing your personal and professional lives, Diana's commitment to what I do here goes a long way toward explaining how it works."

"You have three children?"

"Yes, and I'm very proud of each one. Jane is a pre-med student at Cornell, Peter is a senior at Canisius High School, and Laura is a freshman in high school. The kids have wide and varied interests, and I try and share in all of them. Every minute that I'm home is spent with my family, and our balance is good." Dr. Caty's eyes were certainly alive with pride. "Buffalo is a wonderful place to raise a family. It's not only a terrific medical community, but I'm able to take advantage of the fact that I can be home to spend time with my children. In some of the bigger cities I might not be able to make things work so easily. I was able to coach my daughter's hockey teams. I'm not sure I would have had such an opportunity in Boston, or Philadelphia, or New York. I thoroughly enjoy Buffalo."

"With all that you have going on, you were able to coach your daughter's hockey team?" I asked in amazement.

"If at the end of the day my kids didn't know me, I would be a failure."

"And being a dad and a surgeon must be difficult, as you get to see the results of children being in an accident. Did you fear for your children as they were growing?"

Dr. Caty shook off the question. "Our children played sports and participated in everything, but the fragility of life is always there in the back of my mind. All parents fear for their children. As parents, Diana and I were no different, and we made sure that the kids didn't take unnecessary risks. We certainly didn't have a trampoline at home, and the children wore their headgear."

"My kids have a trampoline," I whispered.

"Get rid of it," Dr. Caty said.

"You spoke of the fragility of life," I said. "When you're talking to parents, how do you answer their questions as to why it happened to them?"

"I try to be supportive, of course, but I'm not in the position to answer questions about what is fair and what isn't. I'm not wise enough to discern God's plan for any of us."

"I find faith to be an interesting aspect of the discussion that I've had with members of the staff," I said. "How does faith enter into your work as a surgeon?"

Dr. Caty contemplated the question for a moment, but provided a detailed answer. "There are a number of ways, actually. As a caretaker for children, I feel that we're here to do God's work. Also, faith plays a huge role in support for families and caregivers. Those families with a strong faith tend to be respectful, and they maintain their dignity. I feel that God is there in the details of what we do. It's definitely helpful when parents believe in a greater good, but personally speaking, faith plays a role in that it makes me do what I do."

"I'm a little uncomfortable with the next question," I said. "But how about children that are victims of abuse? Is it difficult to work through anger in such a situation?"

"I don't feel anger," Dr. Caty said. "I'm not in the position to judge other people. Personally, I'm very uncomfortable in judging others. Besides, when you hate, where do you draw the line?"

I must have looked confused because Dr. Caty quickly clarified it for me. "Do you judge it as abuse if someone leaves cleaning solution out that a child can get into? Do I judge someone who puts a trampoline up in their backyard?"

I turned my head away as I thought about my children jumping on the trampoline.

"I certainly seek to understand," Dr. Caty said. "But I have a tendency to look at the positive of a situation rather than being negative. I have a responsibility to try and understand my patients, but I don't judge them. It's not up to me."

"The staff members that I've spoken with, from Brian Smistek to Sister Brenda, to Ellen Eckhardt, to Cheryl Klass, are all extremely upbeat," I said. "I'm sure that there are hundreds of others at The Women & Children's Hospital who have a similar attitude."

"We have a terrific staff," Dr. Caty said. "I'm also convinced the happiest people I know provide a service for other people. There are certain motivations in this job that are pretty difficult to ignore. You look at a mother that has to care for a child, at home, around the clock. It's fairly easy to be motivated when you meet someone with that much courage."

I immediately thought of Trina Stinson and all of the other parents who were in a similar situation. I recalled a day earlier in the year when Dr. Caty, fresh out of surgery, attended a Family-Centered Care meeting at eight o'clock at night. "Your dedication to the hospital is unbelievable," I said. When I brought up his attendance at the meeting, Dr. Caty waved me off.

"If you're going to go swimming, you might as well get wet," he said. "There really is no sense in doing something halfway, or just sticking your toe in. I'm committed to the hospital, as many people on the staff are, and I recognize when something is important. The families who are a part of the Family-Centered Care initiative are the important members. Their input can make a difference, and I certainly appreciate anyone who is willing to give of themselves in such a manner."

I was beginning to understand why staff members, as well as patient families, raved about Dr. Caty's communication skills. I was as comfortable speaking with him as I would be speaking to my best friend. The next question that floated into my mind came out of nowhere but was a natural progression of the interview. "What about those people who do not live up to your high standards? You demand a lot of yourself. How do you handle it when a staff member is not pulling his or her own weight?"

"Again, it's about judging others," Dr. Caty began. "If I'm to demand excellence of myself while I'm doing my job, then I'm being counter-productive if I dress down an employee or belittle a resident. I certainly expect anyone associated with the department to do the very best that they can, but we all need to be responsible for ourselves to a certain extent."

Dr. Caty's response to the question was certainly in line with his philosophy of helping others. I had entered the interview searching for the spirit of the man, and having had a child who had been a patient, I was not surprised by what I was finding out, but Dr. Caty's outlook was refreshing.

"We have spoken today about general concerns, motivations, and overall impressions. Everything that we've talked about falls in line with how you are perceived as a successful surgeon and a humanist. How does it all come together here to make a patient's stay comfortable?"

"Its really about respect," Dr. Caty said. "When I went through medical school, the training was so difficult. We were overworked and sleep deprived. It gets to you and it can dehumanize you if you let it. I remember growing up and really absolutely loving ice hockey, and then when my family and I made a trip to the Hockey Hall of Fame, I realized I didn't know ten years of players because they had played when I was training. My point is that you can get lost in this field and lose your connection with people. I have been able to stay balanced by asking myself how I would want to be treated if I were sick and lonely. My training has allowed me to be a resource for my patients and the people that I see on a daily basis. I need to use what God has given to me as a resource. I owe that much to my patients, my family, and to myself."

I was nearly too stunned to speak. Dr. Caty's words were more inspirational than I could put into words. I wondered about how different the world might be if we all saw things through his tired eyes.

Before I had the chance to ask the final question, Dr. Caty continued. "I'm an optimist," he said. "I'm here to offer hope, and when someone does something for me, I like to say thanks a lot. It doesn't take much time or trouble to treat others with respect."

I thought back to how Dr. Caty greeted me. *So good to see you.* Just five simple words, but completely in line with everything else we had discussed.

"What makes The Women & Children's Hospital of Buffalo work?"

"Passion," Dr. Caty said without hesitation. "There's not much done around here without great passion."

Realizing I was taking up much more time than I ever dreamed possible, I ended the interview, explaining I would like to discuss even more if we had the chance. I shook Dr. Caty's hand, and he didn't disappoint. "Thanks a lot," he said.

As I headed down in the elevator, I thought about my impression of Dr. Michael Caty on the day when he discussed how Jacob's surgery had gone. I had known all I needed to know about the man; he was driven in his work; proud of the accomplishments of the hospital; and ultimately immersed in the business of helping children.

Later in the day, I stepped out into the bright sunshine of a beautiful fall day. I lingered at the front entrance to the hospital as I tried to understand how I could incorporate a bit of Dr. Caty's attitude into my own daily existence. I gathered my notebooks and headed for a picnic table. A young mother and a child walked down the sidewalk on the Hodge Street side of the hospital. It seemed to me that the beautiful, blond haired, blue-eyed boy was struggling with the idea of seeing his doctor. His mother was bent to his ear, whispering words of encouragement. I wondered if either the mother or the child knew how lucky they were to be entering such an institution where Dr. Caty and a staff of wonderful people were so passionate about being human.

CHAPTER 11

The Story of Olivia Stockmeyer
Part III

"Where there is great love, there are always miracles."
—Willa Cather

Kim and Kevin Stockmeyer were feeling that they were trapped in a nightmare that wasn't easy to shake. Friday turned to Saturday, but neither parent felt the least bit rested. Just 24 hours earlier, they didn't know anything about pulmonary edema, but Saturday greeted them with another new word.

"The doctors took a another chest X-ray and found that Olivia had a pneumothorax, which is a hole in her lung," Kim said. "It was causing air to escape into her chest cavity. The doctor explained that these holes usually heal on their own and that Olivia's body would absorb the air."

"Yet the real terror in the situation is that you don't exactly know what is happening. The uncertainty and the unknown drives you crazy," Kevin added. "We were simply of the mindset that Olivia would be just fine in a short period of time, but we had just had our world completely turned upside down so we were pretty unstable."

"We were dealing with shock," Kim said. "We were overtired, and we were real confused, but the staff at the hospital kept us pointed forward. They were straightforward in their assessment and they did their best to keep us informed. Olivia was doing okay, but she still required oxygen. She was removed from the bi-pap machine because they didn't want to force air into her lungs so that the hole could repair. Olivia was on a regular oxygen mask."

"And man, did she fight that," Kevin said. "She was in arm restraints, but she kept ripping at the mask."

"We had to get up every ten or fifteen minutes to adjust the mask," Kim said. "Not only was Olivia uneasy, but we felt as if we were going out of our minds."

"Still, we felt as though her body was healing and we knew enough to try and stay strong," Kevin said. "We stayed at the hospital all day, of course, but we had dinner together and vowed to get through it a moment at a time."

"And that's when I broke down," Kim said. "It was such a strange situation. Olivia was stable, and although she was fighting with the mask, she was doing fine. I sat at her bedside, with Kevin right there beside me, and I just started to cry. Kevin looked at me a little strangely, and I shrugged my shoulders and told him that I had no idea why I was crying, but that this time, I was the one who was certain that something wasn't quite right."

"I figured that Kim was just tired and that the best thing she could do was head home and get some rest," Kevin said. "After all, we had been at it since early Friday morning. We certainly weren't going to get a good night's sleep, but we needed to be away."

On Saturday night, Kim's father stayed at the bedside. "Olivia's breathing stats actually improved overnight," Kim explained, "but they worsened again in the early morning by the time I arrived at the hospital."

Both Kim and Kevin showed considerable discomfort in explaining what happened next. Just as they were getting used to the idea that the typically routine surgery had left Olivia straining to breathe, they were not blaming anyone or anything. Instead, they were facing the situation head-on, practically, intelligently, and in constant communication with the hospital staff. They were looking forward to the moment when everything would be better again. They anticipated the moment when they would walk through the hospital doors with their baby healthy again. It didn't quite happen that way.

"I was holding Olivia in a chair beside the bed," Kim said. "Olivia wasn't exactly calm, but she felt so good in my arms. I was actually cherishing every second of it, but Olivia's nurse for the day stopped by to see us and became instantly alarmed by Olivia's labored breathing. Yet the staff had continued to do chest X-rays and it was apparent that there wasn't any more air accumulating."

"We all believed that the pneumothorax was healing or that it had completely healed," Kevin said. All at once, he became reflective. "The worst thing about being in that situation is that you want it to be all better, right now. There's no doubt that either one of us would have switched places with Olivia. We just felt so helpless."

"We all felt that we were doing what needed to be done, but it was going to take time, and that was something that was difficult to understand," Kim explained.

"And time moves so slowly," Kevin added. "It felt a lot like being in purgatory must feel like."

The couple did not just sit idly by. Instead, Kim and Kevin began to monitor all of Olivia's vital signs on their own. "It's hard to take your eyes away from the beeping monitors," Kim said. "You don't know what all of it means, but you start looking for benchmarks."

"I was absolutely obsessed with Olivia's respiratory rate," Kevin said. "The staff continued to do all that they could, and there weren't any accumulating fluids, but that rate just seemed wrong. I paced the room and mentioned her respiratory rate every three seconds. I just couldn't take my eyes off of it."

"That's when I turned his advice back on him," Kim said. "Kevin was going to spend Sunday night at the hospital, so I pushed him out the door and told him to get some rest. My family was with me, and we were just looking at the monitors. Kevin needed rest."

"That car ride from Buffalo to Amherst was so strange," Kevin said. "I was painfully tired, and mentally drained, but I can remember thinking how weird it was that life was still going on even though we were in such a horrible situation. What I would have given to just have a normal Sunday, you know?"

At precisely the time that Kevin was walking through the front door of his home alone, Kim was back at the hospital, searching for answers. "My grandmother had recently passed away, and in a quiet moment my mother said, 'Mom, if there's anything you can do…'" Kim bowed her head as she spoke. She was having trouble believing how the entire situation played out. "I had a good Catholic upbringing," Kim said, "but I never truly considered myself religious or anything. That's why my searching out Chaplain Betty was so strange. It was almost as if my grandmother had asked me to seek out Chaplain Betty to bless Olivia and say a prayer with us. Chaplain Betty was unbelievably comforting, and it felt good to know that I had another ally in the fight."

Yet Kevin's obsession with Olivia's monitors was right on the mark. As Kevin telephoned his mother from the comfort of his home, Olivia's respiratory rate increased. The nurse, Val, quickly alerted attending physician, Dr. Budi.

"Dr. Budi explained that they were going to have to put Olivia on a ventilator," Kim said. "He explained that Olivia needed assistance to breath. He asked us to step out of the room for about twenty minutes or so."

Kim's heart was racing. She had the presence of mind to ask her mother to place a call to Kevin.

"You can't imagine what it felt like to have a call come in while I was talking to my mother," Kevin explained. "When I heard Kim's mother on the line, my heart nearly stopped. Kim's mother explained what happened, and before I even had the chance to digest the information, I was back on the line with my mother, just screaming that Olivia was in real trouble. The worst drive of my life had been the commute from the hospital back to the empty house, but let me tell you, this was about a thousand times more difficult."

Kim and her family walked right by the PICU waiting room

and instead headed for the empty surgical waiting room. "There were people in the PICU waiting room," Kim explained, "and I just didn't feel like being around strangers. The worst part was not knowing what was happening in ICU. Every second passed like a month, and I was in a state of absolute panic. I was crying, shaking, and dry-heaving. My family was trying to comfort me, but of course, I was thinking the worst."

Kim's nightmare continued to grow. "While we were waiting another mother walked by the waiting room. The woman's child was also in the PICU, just a few beds away from Olivia. When the woman passed the room, I caught her eyes. We never spoke a single word, but in her eyes I saw all that I needed to see. We were both mothers of sick children, but at that precise moment, that anonymous woman was feeling sorry for me. The look on her face sent me into a dizzying spin that was compounded by the fact that doctors were soon being paged to the PICU, stat!"

Kevin was racing back to the hospital. "I have no idea how fast I was going," Kevin said. "Let's just say that I was a tad over the speed limit."

"I couldn't bring myself to return to the PICU," Kim said. "With what was happening all around me, I didn't think that I could take even the sight of Olivia or what was happening to her. Finally, my mother went into the PICU, and the first thing she heard was a nurse on the telephone saying that they needed other doctors and surgeons to the PICU immediately. "The patient's name is Stockmeyer," Kim's mother heard.

"My mother shouted that Olivia was her granddaughter and she asked what was happening. The nurse just said that Olivia wasn't doing very well at the moment."

As Kim told the story, her eyes filled with tears. It was apparent that her heart was breaking all over again. "I wasn't in control of anything," Kim explained. "My body took the news as a personal attack and I was physically sick into one of the garbage cans in the waiting room."

"That's precisely when I walked in," Kevin said. "I saw Kim with her family, and the whole world stopped. My mind was screaming at me that my beautiful little girl had died. I just lost it. I didn't have any information at all, but I was sure that I knew what had happened."

Before Kevin could find out exactly what was happening, Chaplain Betty returned. Her mere presence was enough to calm the shocked family for just a moment. "Chaplain Betty had left the floor," Kim said. "Something made her come back to our floor. We'll never really know why she returned, but I was so glad to see her. I immediately asked if we could go to the PICU."

"Of course, you can," Chaplain Betty said. "You're the parents."

"It was an absolute mob scene in the room," Kevin said. "There were at least ten doctors working on our daughter."

"Val caught our attention and signaled to us that they were nearly finished and asked us to stay back for just a few more minutes," Kim said.

The young couple watched the scene realizing that everything in their lives was leading up to that very moment. "There's not a coherent thought in your head. You're just looking for something, anything to hold onto, and there's nothing there," Kevin said.

The commotion in the room appeared to die down. "As I think back on it, it was amazing to watch the teamwork," Kim said. "Of course, I wasn't thinking that at the time, but I thank God every night for everyone that was in that room that afternoon."

Dr. Budi approached Kim and Kevin.

"Dr. Budi explained that the pneumothorax had not healed and that the air had been collecting in between her lung and heart rather than her lung and the chest wall. That was why the X-rays hadn't shown an accumulation of air."

"We knew it was bad," Kevin said, "but we certainly weren't prepared for what he said next. Dr. Budi explained that the air collected in her chest cavity had caused her lungs to collapse and that she went into cardiac arrest."

"There is no way that a parent should have to hear that their child is in cardiac arrest," Kim said as the tears returned to her eyes. "Dr. Budi explained that Olivia needed epinephrine to keep her heart pumping. He said that they had placed emergency chest tubes to release the air from her chest cavity. Dr. Budi said that Olivia was also on an oscillating ventilator that provided short puffs of air so that her lungs didn't fully expand and the pneumothorax could heal. He said that if Olivia's condition didn't improve that she would need to be placed on an ECMO machine. I asked him what ECMO was and he said that it would pump her blood and breathe for her. I asked him if he meant life support, and he said yes."

Kim had heard enough. Her mind threatened to shut down, but just as she thought she couldn't take anymore, Kevin asked one more question. "Is this machine something that she can come off of?"

Dr. Budi's eyes filled with tears, and he looked away from Kevin and Kim. "I'm sorry," he said.

CHAPTER 12

The Story of Joanne Lana & Stone's Buddies

"You're Never Alone."
—*Stone's Buddies Motto*

"The great lesson is that the sacred is in the ordinary,
that it is to be found in one's daily life,
in one's neighbors, friends, and family,
in one's backyard."
—*Abraham Maslow*

Joanne Lana moved through the halls of the Women & Children's Hospital of Buffalo at about a thousand miles per hour. As the program coordinator for the patient family program known simply as Stone's Buddies, Joanne doesn't understand the meaning of standing still, or waiting for life to come to her. She smiled hurriedly as we met in the middle of a crowded cafeteria. It was just a little before noon, but Joanne wasn't interested in lunch. "I have about 45 minutes," she said. "I'm sorry, but there's so much going on lately."

Before we even had the chance to settle in, Joanne handed me a Stone's Buddies backpack. "I figured that it would be easier to tell you what we're all about by showing you the packet that we welcome our members with."

I opened up the pack that has the Stone's Buddies logo emblazoned across the front. It is a bright red and yellow logo with the silhouetted figures of a child on a swing and an adult behind the child, guiding the swing. Inside the pack are a variety of special items, including a Stone's Buddies T-shirt, pillowcase, stress ball, bandanna, glow-in-the-dark bracelet, and a hefty guide to help families cope with their child's hospitalization.

"The program was started in September of 2005. It was created in the memory of former Women & Children's patient Stone Filipovich. Did you know of Stone?"

"Yes," I said. "I heard Stone's story on the radio."

"Everyone in Western New York knew Stone," Joanne said with a smile. "He was an amazing little boy."

The Story of Stone Filipovich

Every moment of every day is worth living, and being able to appreciate that fact is the first step toward being alive and well instead of being alive but sick. Stone's life is evidence of that. At four years of age, Stone had spent more than half of his life fighting an aggressive brain tumor. He was a real trooper who never stopped smiling despite countless tests, surgeries, medical therapies, and unimaginable pain. Stone's body was sick, but his spirit was so alive that it energized everyone who was lucky enough to meet him. From the comfort of his mother's arms, Stone often assured his loved ones that he was "okay" despite the fact that he knew differently. The big heart beating inside his little chest would let him do nothing less.

Although Stone's life touched more hearts than most who live ten times as long as he did, it's not just the battle he waged for life that inspired so many. Early in 2004, Stone became known to many throughout Western New York during the annual KISS Cares for Kids Radio-thon to benefit The Women and Children's Hospital of Buffalo. Stone and his family demonstrated extraordinary courage while sharing their stories, experiences, and feelings with host Janet Snyder and Nicholas Picholas.

During that radio performance, Stone ignored the aches and pains that were his daily companions to project his small voice over the airwaves, and his words forever changed the lives of those who heard his story of courage.

Although Stone's life ended shortly after his fourth birthday in 2004, his inspiring spirit was strong enough to make an impact through Stone's Buddies by reminding others like him that they are not alone.

"It was important to our family as we coped with Stone's illness that we were not alone in fighting his condition," said Stone's mother Roberta. "From the beginning, we felt an overwhelming sense of support from the doctors, nurses and other families who were fighting similar battles every day. That's why we feel it's so important and we are proud to know that Stone's memory will continue to help other children and families at Women & Children's Hospital."

Roberta is also very giving as she explains the Pennies From Stone aspect of Stone's Buddies. The information below is written on The Women & Children's Hospital of Buffalo web page:

According to Stone's mom, Stone is forever sending tiny reminders that he is watching over them by dropping pennies from Heaven where she can find them. From the earliest days of his diagnosis with a brain tumor, Stone's tiny hand was often seen wrapped tightly around a fistful of pennies. He loved coins and collected them faithfully every day, depositing each coin in his piggy bank for the rainy day he knew would come in the future.

When Stone left this Earth, Stone's mom believes that—somehow—he took his special treasure with him. Every time that Stone's mom finds a precious penny, she knows it's a priceless reminder of the love she shared with Stone and his assurance that she will never be alone.

Stone Filipovich was an inspiration to all, and remains as such, even in death. He never fully realized his dream of riding his grandfather's Harley-Davidson motorcycle, but through his short life, he allows the dreams of others to remain alive.

★   ★   ★

"Everyone knew about Stone," Joanne said. "He's still so alive in the halls of this hospital."

"How many children are a part of Stone's Buddies?" I asked.

"Too many," Joanne said. "About one hundred children are enrolled. Approximately twenty-five percent of those kids have brain tumors. It's a club that no child wants to be a member of, but we help each other to make it through."

"Tell me about yourself," I said.

Joanne looked perplexed with the idea of speaking about herself. "It's all about the program," she answered. "But if I must bring myself into it, I'd have to say that I have the best job in the world. Every day is different and hour-to-hour I'm not real sure what direction I'll be heading in. It's the perfect job for me because I suffer from adult attention deficit disorder." Joanne laughed heartily. "Seriously, I need to be able to adapt to changing situations. I guess that's true of a lot of people who work here, but I have to be ready for anything."

Joanne glanced at her watch quickly, but her eyes danced as she described what might happen in a "typical" day. "I start the day no later than 5 a.m. I have four children, so those early morning hours are spent running on the treadmill, doing a few loads of laundry, cleaning up, and getting the kids off to school. Once I get to work, I check e-mails and telephone messages. The messages that I might get allow me to assemble my day. There may be one of the Stone's Buddies members in the hospital, and if that is the case, I'll stop by and visit with them. I may also get a call from the Child Life Department letting me know that there is a child who is appropriate for inclusion in the program."

Joanne paused for a long moment and I realized that she was thinking about a very sick child who may be enrolled in the program. I could tell that something that she said aloud stirred a responsibility in her mind. "The people in the community are also hugely supportive," she said finally. "We involve our children in special events and fund-raisers. For instance, Wal-Mart works with us by adopting a Stone's Buddies child for each of their store locations. People in the community tend to be much more supportive when they can put a face to a cause."

On cue, Joanne slid three collections of photos across the table. One of the photos was a thank-you to a local car dealership. It showed fourteen shots of Stone's Buddies members in a variety of poses. Some of the children had shaved heads, others were posed with sports stars, and still others were doing arts and crafts. I stared at the photograph for a long moment, finally focusing on the image of two young boys who were no older than five. Each child's head was shaved and there were serious looks covering their faces.

"There must be a lot of sadness," I muttered.

Joanne answered with a smile. "Oh, I cry," she said. "But, you know, I've never had to answer the question, 'Why me?' I am blessed to be able to meet all of the families and to be a part of their amazing strength of character."

The next set of images was a thank-you to the Buffalo Sabres Hockey Team. Seven of the Sabres players were posed next to the Stone's Buddies children. The children were posing with shirts, and drawings that they created with the help of the players. In each of the sixteen photographs there was at least one smiling child.

"We love when the sports teams visit," Joanne said. "It gives the children quite a lift. The Bills and the Sabres have been great."

The final sheet of photos was a thank you to one of the high school classes in Western New York. My eyes were drawn to a girl who was no older than three years of age. "God, they're so beautiful," I whispered.

Joanne laughed. "See, you're ready to help in the program. It's pretty hard to stay sad when you're around children doing fun activities. Every once in awhile I'll attend a Bills or Sabres game with some of the children, and it is such a blast seeing them outside the hospital setting, having such a wonderful time. The players and the coaches are very generous when it comes to arranging seating for Stone's Buddies."

Joanne did not allow me to linger too long on the faces of the children. She handed me a massive book entitled, *One Step at a*

Time. "It's important for the family members to know they are not alone either," Joanne said. "This is a practical guide that will assist family members to ask the right questions."

The cover of the book featured the words hope, trust, inspiration, encourage, and comfort. Joanne observed me reading the words, and she flashed a hopeful smile.

"That is what we are all about," she said. "Our goal is to be a beacon of light for surviving one of the most difficult of life's experiences."

As Joanne glanced at her watch once more, I realized that it was time for me to leave. I picked up Stone's bandanna and my mind drifted back to the sound of his voice as it came through my car radio shortly before his death. Stone had spoken of hope and love and family. His message lived on in the development of the program established in his honor.

Joanne was nearly giddy with excitement as she walked away. "I'm going to visit with one of the members of Stone's Buddies," she said. "I just love these kids."

Before I could even formulate a reply, Joanne was off and racing through the halls of the hospital. It came to mind that she loved her job because of the simple fact that she was doing God's work.

CHAPTER 13

The Story of Anthony Stinson
Part III

"To be alive, to be able to see, to walk—it's all a miracle.
I have adopted the technique of living life
from miracle to miracle."
—Arthur Rubenstein

A prolonged hospital stay of a child is absolute misery for every member of the family. The outside world has a tendency to fade into the background as the mother, father, and grandparents spend their days in chairs beside the bed or in waiting rooms. Every waking moment is spent in the discomfort of not knowing what will happen next, or debating the advantage of having another cup of coffee. Lifelong sleeping and eating habits are strewn aside, and the fatigue felt in the minds and bodies of those involved is extremely sharp. In the case of Anthony Stinson and his family, all of those discomforts were compounded with the fact that there was a good chance that Anthony would never be the same again.

"I was so hopeful," Trina Stinson explained. She was seated on the bed next to her son as she told the story nearly four years later. "My mind was playing tricks on·me, but I just didn't think that Anthony would suffer from a lifelong affliction. I did not have a lot of information on what we were dealing with because it was such an unusual case. I firmly believed that on the day when they would lighten up on Anthony's medicine that he would spring to life and greet me with all of the enthusiasm of his earlier days."

A week had passed since Anthony's devastating seizure. The staff prepared to extubate Anthony, and Trina waited, as hopeful as she had been prior to Anthony's birth. "It felt as if he were being delivered to me for a second time. I went to sleep in the PICU parent room, but I remember asking the nurse to wake me up immediately when Anthony's eyes started to open."

Trina bowed her head to the carpet, as if she could find some answer for her disappointment in the shag of the rug. "I wanted Anthony to know that his mommy was there. I needed him to feel that everything would be okay."

The nurse nudged Trina out of her fitful sleep to explain that Anthony was waking up.

"I ran over to Anthony's bed, and ever so slowly, his eyes opened, but Anthony did not look at me and smile. He didn't say my name or ask for a drink of water. Instead, his eyes were completely vacant, and he looked right through me as though I weren't even there. It wasn't because of his vision problems. It was because Anthony had suffered extensive brain damage."

Trina's face adopted a look as though she were watching a ten-car accident. She tried hard to force a smile through, but the devastation was undeniable.

"I can remember the voice in my head just screaming at me. He woke up! He's supposed to be better! He's supposed to walk with me! He's supposed to talk to me! He's supposed to ask for Nicholas!"

Trina leaned into the bed. She touched her son lightly, and I assumed that she needed to feel connected to him somehow.

"I just didn't understand. We had a new Anthony, and it broke my heart to understand that this once energetic boy, who had a powerful zest for life and loved to make other people laugh, was now a child that had lost every single ability that he ever had."

Trina's eyes did a quick dance across the chalkboard directly across from the bed. When she became convinced of the fact that she did not need to administer care to Anthony at the moment, her thoughts returned to that most lonely of days.

"I remember seeing the neurologist, Dr. Patricia Duffner. She had been on duty all through that first week. She had seen Anthony walking and talking one day, and in the PICU the next. Dr. Duffner was just astonished at what had happened. I swear, she was as devastated by what had happened as I was. Dr. Duffner checked Anthony's EEG's from April 18th and April 19th, and his MRI's from April 18th and April 22nd. She explained that they were dramatically different and that she didn't truly have an explanation as to why."

Trina's thought patterns shifted and I saw the palpable difference in her demeanor as she stopped talking about Anthony's care for a moment and concentrated on the care she received at the hospital. "Dr. Duffner stopped by to see Anthony every single day. Even if she wasn't on duty, she stopped by. I'm talking even on the weekends! It was more than just her job. Dr. Duffner knew what kind of shape I was in, and she realized that I just needed to see her. I needed to speak to her every day. I needed to be reassured. I needed her comforting words to get through another hour, another day, another week. After Anthony was discharged, Dr. Duffner allowed me to bring him to her clinic every single week until I felt comfortable. After a few months, we went every two weeks, then monthly, then every other month. It has now been four-and-a-half years and we see Dr. Sarah Finnegan every two or three months. I must say that Dr. Finnegan is every bit as wonderful as Dr. Duffner."

For the very first time, as Trina spoke about the wonderful compassion of the neurologist, I saw through her mask of bravery. "Dr. Duffner is a wonderful woman who brought me through it. I'm telling you, for the next four months, she answered every single one of my questions. She addressed all of my worries, told me what diseases they were testing for, and above all else, she comforted me as a human being."

During those four months, the Stinson family dynamic was severely altered. Trina, Tom, Nicholas, and Anthony were forced to enter a completely new world fraught with extensive medical testing, therapy, insurance claims and denials, as all the while they fought for normalcy.

"Nicholas was almost four years old when Anthony got sick, and I must say that he was unbelievably strong."

As Trina spoke of Nicholas, she glanced over her shoulder, but Nicholas was out of hearing distance in the other room. "Tom and I took turns staying with Anthony at the hospital so that each child was always with one parent or the other. Nick visited with Anthony at the hospital for a little while every single day." Trina's voice dropped an octave. "Can you imagine how it feels for a brother to see his little buddy in such a condition?"

Trina's question ripped through my own body. I thought of my sons and their relationship to one another. My mind threatened to explode in a shattering of tears, but I simply nodded.

"It absolutely *killed* me to know that other people were taking care of Nicholas while I was at the hospital. My life was falling apart, but I was motivated only by what I needed to do for each of my children."

Out of the corner of my eye, I saw Nicholas approaching the room once more. I wasn't sure if he knew that his mother was speaking of his relationship with his brother. I turned to Nicholas and he smiled as brightly as his mother. Seeing Nicholas stirred all of the emotions that I was feeling up to that point. I reached for a glass of water and sipped it slowly as I paged through a medical summary written by Trina in an effort to get help for Anthony. The letter was written in 2004. I read it quickly as Trina and Nicholas shared a moment together.

> *To Whom it May Concern:*
>
> *Hello, my name is Trina Stinson. I have put together this packet on my son, Anthony Stinson. He is a 4-year-old boy who started his life as a healthy baby. The older he got, the less healthy he became.*
>
> *On April 19, 2002, at 22 months old, Anthony went into status epilepticus. His genetics doctor thought that his diagnosis*

was possibly Leigh Syndrome, or subacute necrotizing encephalomyelopathy. This was based on the clinical course and the findings of the MRI on 04/22/02 of areas of edema in the thalami and caudate heads, although a secondary effect of prolonged seizure activity with edema could not be ruled out. So, at this time, Anthony is not diagnosed and is a completely different child. Here are some of the things that Anthony has to deal with on a daily basis:

- *Gasric-Jejunal continuous feeding*
- *Tracheal Laryngeal Diversion*
- *Chronic Lung Disease*
- *Always uncomfortable*
- *Seizure disorder*
- *Gastrointestinal Reflux*
- *Digital stimulation for bowel movements*
- *Select immune deficiency/receives monthly IV therapy*
- *Has been medically unstable since 04/19/02*
- *Oxygen required 24 hours per day*
- *Frequent suctioning*
- *Legally blind*
- *24-hour monitoring for heart rate and oxygen levels*
- *20 hours of nursing care required*
- *15 different medicines; 29 times a day*
- *Respiratory vest, chest PT and cough assist treatments every 4 hours*
- *Relies on parent, nurses, and therapists for his every day needs*
- *Cannot sit, stand, or talk, although he can be calmed by his parent and regular nurses, and does try to move his head when spoken to. He has no head control and very little volitional movement. He stretches, raises arm in discomfort, moves when his feet are tickled, and sometimes hits a switch toy when playing with therapists.*
- *Receives occupational therapy, physical therapy, vision therapy, speech therapy, special education and massage therapy weekly. 16 visits per week.*

- *Countless doctor appointments.*
- *Only supportive care, not curative.*

Although it has been over 2 years since Anthony got sick, we are still desperately trying to find out our son's diagnosis. We realize that he cannot be what he was without a miracle, but if there is something that can medically stabilize him and make him comfortable, he can have the quality of life that he deserves.

If you can take the time to go through our son's life story and possibly come up with something, or know someone else who may be able to help, we would greatly appreciate it, and happily pay whatever fee you may require.

Thank you for taking the time to at least read this letter.
Respectfully,
Thomas, Trina and Nicholas Stinson
Loving and devoted family to Anthony Stinson

I folded the letter closed in front of me. Nicholas and Trina's attention was on Anthony as mother and son laughed about something that had happened in Nicholas' day. When Trina turned back to me, her smile was firmly in place. "Are you ready to talk about when Anthony finally came home?" she asked.

"If my heart can take it," I said. In front of me was a thirty-or forty-page document that had a title page stating, *"Medical Summaries on our son. We are desperately searching for a diagnosis and hopefully a cure."*

"It wasn't the easiest transition in the world," Trina said. "I was deathly afraid of having Anthony come home, but home is where he belonged."

CHAPTER 14

The Story of Barb Kourkounis & Family-Centered Care

"The things that matter most in our lives
are not fantastic or grand.
They are the moments when we touch one another."
—*Jack Kornfield, Buddhist Monk, Author & Teacher*

My stomach flutters each and every time I walk through the doors of The Women & Children's Hospital of Buffalo. Of course the fluttering is a direct result of my child having to undergo a lengthy surgery, but it is also in direct response to the parents and children who are entering those doors for the first time. As I entered the side door on Hodge Street, I stepped out of the way to allow a young mother to walk inside with two boys, who at a passing glance appeared to be identical twins. Each of the boys had a bright red ski cap and a wide smile. Each child stood no higher than three feet tall. I smiled as I held the door and the mother glanced my way, and offered a hurried word of thanks.

Immediately, my mind shifted to the Family-Centered Care initiative and the champion of the cause, Barb Kourkounis. I was a few minutes late for my appointment to speak with Barb, but given her passion for the cause, I'm certain she would have wanted me to hold the door open for the young family. The mission of the committee is to bring a family perspective to the healthcare experience in order to meet the needs of patients and families of The Women and Children's Hospital of Buffalo, through exceptional care, communication, education and research.

Barb and I settled in a quiet corner of the busy cafeteria. I sipped from a cup of coffee, but Barb didn't need any of the artificial energy. She was as prepared and passionate as she seemed to be each time I met her. She was also coming off of a couple of very difficult days because her husband Jim was recovering from surgery at Buffalo General Hospital. Still, Barb appeared rested, and I didn't have to say much in the way of greeting to prompt her discussion of her work.

"Why did I become a nurse?" Barb began. "I suppose that, to be perfectly honest, there were few options for a young woman back in 1968. My choices were to get married or become a secretary, teacher, or nurse. My mother, Jessie, and my sister, Winkie, were nurses, so it was a fairly natural step. A career in computers was a bizarre option back then. I do remember that someone came to the door one time to try to sell my father on getting his daughter into computers, but my father would have nothing of it."

Barb's eyes danced back to the day when she decided to become a nurse. "I suppose that I am who I am today because of my father, Ferdinand. He was a laborer, a painter, and a union steward. He had a real passion for rooting for the underdog. Even when he was rooting for sports teams, he always pulled for the underdog. My dad helped out at our church, although he seldom attended Sunday service, and he was always helping his neighbors. He had a tremendous work ethic too."

"You're close with your dad?" I asked with a smile.

"He passed when I was a rebellious 16-year-old," Barb answered, "but, yes, I saw in him the joy and satisfaction that comes from helping others. His deeds were never fantastic or grand, but he obviously touched people because he was loved by many."

I searched my mind for one of my set questions, but Barb was so well prepared that she didn't wait for the question.

"I've always been a critical care nurse. For years I thought that emergency and intensive care were the greatest challenges and would be the most rewarding. You know, the greatest satisfaction in doing my job doesn't come from any sort of technical expertise. There are nurses who take great pride in doing the technical aspect of their jobs well, but I am satisfied in my work when I'm able to put patients and families at ease. I want them to feel comfort in my presence. I feel good when I am able to help them cope when the odds are against them. I think that this is what makes me passionate about my work."

"Rooting for the underdog," I whispered.

"The thing is, when I began my career it was a completely different world. I worked at the Chaffee Hospital in Springville from 1974 through 1990. In those days, the doctors weren't in the emergency room. The nurse was the first line of defense. I was a night supervisor as well as an ER nurse. I learned so much at Chaffee. That was when it became apparent to me that the most important aspect of my job was in dealing with the families."

Barb didn't hesitate. She took me back through the years to one of the stories that helped shape her bulldog determination to spearhead the Family Care initiative at The Women & Children's Hospital of Buffalo.

"One night at Chaffee, I was in the ER alone when someone rang the doorbell. Believe it or not, that's how you got into the ER in those days." Barb smiled wistfully, but her mind quickly turned back to that fateful night. "I opened the door to find a father standing there with a boy of about thirteen slung up over his shoulder. The boy looked nearly dead and he was barely breathing. I later learned that he had severe asthma and chronic lung disease, and that he was scheduled for admission to CHOB for experimental treatment.

"I grabbed a resuscitation bag and placed the mask on the boy's face. I placed the dad's hands on the bag and mask and showed him what he had to do while I made a quick phone call for help. The doctor lived close by and was there quickly, but despite all of our efforts, the boy passed. About six months later, I was in the grocery store when the father came walking toward me. He extended his hand and said, 'I want to thank you for allowing me to participate in trying to save my child's life'."

Barb's passion for the Family-Centered Care initiative is legendary to all members of the parent advisory council. "Being a nurse at Chaffee left us little choice. For years there was no in-house staff. This was a small rural hospital where nurses evaluated the ER patients, then called the doctor, either in their office or at home. Families were never sent to the waiting room. They were at their loved one's side providing support, assisting with care, answering and asking questions. This was sometimes a bit challenging, but patients and families seemed more satisfied with their medical care then."

I recognized Barb's words as the spoken model for the Family-Centered Care initiative that we spoke about at the monthly meetings.

"One of my most difficult days was when I escorted a father to the morgue. This poor man was out of town when his wife and children died in a traffic accident. I went with him to the morgue so that he could say goodbye to his family."

I felt a bit of fluttering in my heart as I considered the fact that Barb actually thrives on being a front-line defense in critical situations. I considered asking her how she can handle the pain associated with her job, but she is off and running before I can formulate the question.

"I think that patients and families feel better when things are done *with* them instead of *to* them," Barb said. "Just last week I was in a patient's room, working with a young boy who's father was exasperated with the thought of another IV line being placed in his child. I was searching for a workable vein, and the father was impatient with the process. He let me know, in no uncertain terms, that I wasn't going to find a vein. So, instead of being confrontational and difficult, I asked the child's dad what he suggested. He thought about it for a long moment, then told me to look in a very awkward location on the back of his son's arm. Of course, there was a nice, big bulging vein there and it worked out fine. I told the child that his father had been right, and had done a good job in finding that vein. Even though it had been tense for a moment, it made me feel great to see the slight smile that broke across the dad's face when I thanked him."

As Barb finished the story, I considered my own involvement in the Family-Centered Care Initiative. As a parent liaison and a member of the Patient & Parent Advisory Council, I am grateful that I've been asked to participate. The program's mission is to foster a partnership with patients and their families and health care providers at all levels to improve the quality of care that they receive.

"Family-Centered Care is so important to all of our tasks," Barb said. "In our day-to-day tasks, we need to approach every single situation with what is best for the patient, not what works better for the system. Allowing that father to assist in the health-care of his child was crucial to him, but it is also so much more than that."

Barb paused for a brief moment, but I sat back, waiting for the example that was about to absolutely blow my mind.

"There was an infant here that was critically ill. Frankie was a little over two weeks old when she was admitted to our PICU, and she was in my care. Her parents were Philippine-Americans, and there were cultural differences. I worked hard to identify what made them feel good, and I did my best to allow them to assist in the care of their child. It's funny because there were a lot of angels involved. I remember that being one of the cultural differences. The family was very centered on angels. The mother loved to bathe her baby. I clearly recall that I would delay giving her her daily bath until her parents were there. We would move the medical equipment aside and her mother would very carefully, and lovingly, wash her. It was a comfort for them in the middle of some very difficult care, but it was a small allowance on our part."

Barb took a deep breath before continuing, and I quickly understood why she had been forced to hesitate.

"It was early on Christmas morning about three weeks after the child was admitted, that she passed, and the parents' reaction was understandably hysterical. We were at our wit's end trying to figure out how we could possibly comfort them. We needed to find a way to help them 'let go'. Considering that the child's mother helped bathe her daughter each and every day, I asked Mom if she wanted to help get her daughter ready. It was a very difficult, messy situation, but together we removed her many tubes, then bathed and dressed little Frankie for the final time. We found a beautiful pink flannel nightgown and wrapped her in a blanket."

A strong case of gooseflesh made its way up and down my arms and across my neck, and I wiped at my arms as Barb continued with the story.

"On that Christmas Day the family met in the room. For hours, the mom, the dad, and the mom's sister passed the baby back and forth. Having held on to hope right up to the very end, they hadn't made even thought about making funeral arrangements. The family decided on a funeral home and I made the call. I explained the situation to the funeral director so that the transition would be smooth. Dad wouldn't give up the baby," Barb said softly. "He cornered me, and screaming hysterically, cried, 'Barb, I trust you, don't make me do this! Just let me take her home! Please, please, Barb, let me take her home, just for a few hours! I want to show her her room, her toys, her family!"

"My God," I whispered. I was losing control of my right hand as I tried to erase the tingling feeling surging through my body.

"With tears streaming down my cheeks, I firmly told the dad that he could not," Barb said. "I finally convinced him that he could walk the child to the door. I met the woman from the funeral home at the hospital entrance when she arrived with the small box. I asked her to put it back in the car so that the family didn't see it. Then I walked with the family through the halls and down the elevator to the front door. Dad put their beautiful little baby in my arms; we all cried and said good-bye."

Barb was extremely calm as she recounted the story. Meanwhile, I was squirming in my seat.

"I, along with a few other nurses and a very special doctor, attended the funeral. The family seemed genuinely comforted in knowing that we all cared deeply. On Christmas Day, one year later, I received a beautiful note of thanks and a glass angel."

I wasn't sure how I was going to be able to come up with the words, but was certain of my question. "How do you handle it emotionally? How can you face the endless parade of sick children?"

"I've never lost my enthusiasm for my job," Barb answered without hesitation. "Working with children and their families is so inspirational and motivating. Listen, it hurts, but life isn't supposed to be perfectly happy. Struggle is a part of life. Injury and illness are a part of life. And even death is a fact of life. My passion to continue doing what I, and many of my coworkers, do comes from knowing that we can make a small contribution by helping children and their families through these realities."

Barb's words were punctuated with the beginning of tears in her eyes. "Children are just so resilient and forgiving. They don't bring with them all of the emotional baggage that many adults do when they are sick. They aren't lying in bed thinking, 'poor me.' They face what they need to face and don't contemplate secondary gain. Their emotions are pure, and you know what they are thinking. Believe me, you know they hate that you gave them pain when you stuck them with a needle. However, a moment later, they may be laughing and giving you a hug. The children allow us to see that purity of emotion that we have lost by just living."

It was such a beautiful statement that I let it linger in my ears for a brief moment, but Barb was already moving on.

"I feel the emotional pain, of course, but there is a consolation in knowing that I *am* feeling that pain. It's time to quit nursing when you are no longer empathetic. I hurt, but it doesn't interfere with what I need to do. The struggles and the pain make you stronger. There's an old Buddhist prayer that says, 'Hearts Heal Stronger in Broken Places.'"

Barb waved at someone across the room but she didn't miss a beat.

"I learned a long time ago not to internalize the pain or wear it on my shirtsleeves so that my co-workers are focusing on me and not on the needs of the patient and family. That's not to say that I don't appreciate a co-worker's hug after I have been with a family who has received bad news, but then it's time to move on. I try to focus on the child who is in the situation, not on my personal life."

"Tell me about your family," I said.

"I've been married to Jim, for thirty-six years," Barb replied. "He's in the hospital now, but he'll be coming home today. He's a hard-working, well-educated man. We have two children, Jason, who is an art handler and a musician, and Jessie, who is a photojournalist. They are very happy, and healthy, and that is what is important, above all else."

It was apparent that Barb's love for her own family was a driving force in her compassion for the family-centered care that she advocates. It is an initiative that finds its expression in compassion and kindness, but I ask an honest, perhaps naïve question.

"What happens when you're dealing with a family member that is full of anger? Perhaps there have been mistakes made in the technical care of the child, and the family is resistant to any sort of comfort that you're offering."

Barb nodded. "Certainly that happens. Things don't always go as intended. No one is perfect, nor does medicine have all of the answers. I find that in those situations it is best to be direct. I don't make excuses for the doctors, or for anyone else, but neither do I place blame. Instead, I try and focus on what needs to be done. I'm not above saying that I'm sincerely sorry for their predicament, but the best thing to do in that situation is to try and focus the negative energy on what we can do from that point on."

Barb's eyes drifted away from me for a long moment. When she spoke again, I quickly realized that she was dreaming of a different sort of healthcare. Her family focused care is not just an idea; it is a way of life for her.

"Imagine what it would be like if you entered the hospital for a same-day surgery and someone greeted you at the door and explained what would be happening to you on that day. It would certainly take all of the guesswork and anxiety out of the situation. I imagine someone well dressed greeting you with all of your information at the ready. The greeter would say, 'Good Morning, Mr. Fazzolari, I know that you're a little anxious this morning, but this is what we are going to do for you today.'"

"That's a great idea," I replied. "But everything is so money-driven. It would be expensive to treat each person like that."

"Money plays a huge part, of course," Barb said. "Yet we have seminars and classes where we explain the right and wrong ways of speaking with families. Just recently, I asked Dr. Erbe if the Patient & Parent Advisory Council could get on the Grand Rounds agenda to present the core concepts of Family-Centered Care and effective communication techniques. Dr. Erbe, who's been here for quite awhile said, 'Isn't it a shame that we have to explain family-centered care to the staff?' It is a shame."

"Back to the cost of such a program," I said. "Isn't it a shame that a hospital such as The Women and Children's Hospital of Buffalo is forced to almost beg for funds when we are able to finance sports teams anytime that there is a slight chance that they are not profitable?"

"That's a difficult question," Barb answered. "But it's all about where people's priorities lie. On the way in this morning I was listening to a newscast about the effort that people are going through to get the latest doll for Christmas. There are parents willing to spend over a hundred dollars for a stuffed toy that you can tickle. Thirty million people watched *Dancing with the Stars* last night. It's all about misplaced priorities."

"It must be frustrating to think that people understand that the work you're doing here is so critically important, but yet, it is something they don't think about all of the time."

"It is frustrating," Barb said. "It's depressing, actually."

"Tell me about your greatest frustration on a day-to-day basis."

"That's pretty easy," Barb said with a smile. "I am most frustrated with people who either accept the status quo, or naysayers who insist that things can't be changed. I'm extremely frustrated by people who are afraid of change."

The program that Barb is championing at the hospital is certainly a driving force in her life. Sitting across from her, I understood she would work as hard as she could to initiate the changes that she and others have envisioned.

"The other frustrating aspect of working day-to-day with a huge staff of people is that there are men and women in all capacities who do not put forth the effort that they should each and every day."

"That's the way it is in every walk of life," I said.

"Yes, of course, it is, but it's frustrating that people don't evaluate if they are happy with their jobs. This is not a place to stay if you're not committed to what you're doing. We have hundreds of wonderful people working here, but one person's job here affects another's. There is a great deal of pride to be taken in every single job. I'm thinking about two members of a transport team for one of the other hospitals when my husband was on the receiving end of the medical system. These two were courteous, smiling, and really hustling. I thanked them for doing their hard work and great attitudes, and they seemed shocked that I had noticed."

"How proud are you of working at the hospital?"

"I'm very proud of the many dedicated workers that we have here. I *will* be very, very proud when we become all that we can become."

"You're always pointed forward," I said.

"We all have to be," Barb said. "Think of Trina Stinson and her son, Anthony. Think about John and Jackie Adamo and their critically ill child, Taylor. John and Jackie are instrumental members of the parent advisory council. I find it so admirable that there are families who are concerned about the care of all children at this hospital. The Adamos are wonderful people. They are able to look beyond their own devastating situation to see what can be done for those who follow them. Taylor Adamo and Anthony Stinson will never live normal lives, but their parents continually advocate for them and others. They, and so many other families like them, are my inspiration." Barb's eyes fill with tears once again. "That is our responsibility here."

Barb looked beyond me once more. Again she gave a slight wave. "There's Dr. Erbe," she said.

I turned in my chair, but Dr. Erbe had moved from sight.

"There's a man," Barb said, "who remembers everyone. He knows their names and their life stories. He's been here for a long time, and maybe he does things the old-fashioned way, but if you want to talk about family-centered care, he's someone we should all aspire to be like."

Barb did the very thing that I was expecting her to do. She emphasized her point by tugging at my heartstrings once more.

"I recently spoke with a mom that told me this story. Over seven years ago, Dr. Erbe, a geneticist, consulted on her twin daughters with cerebral palsy. She unbelievably also had another child who passed away due to a congenital heart defect. Well, two years ago, the mother returned to the hospital with her twins and ran into Dr. Erbe in one of the elevators. Dr. Erbe recognized the woman, asked how her children were doing, and three days later, sent a card to the mother saying how great it was to see her again and that he was glad that they were doing well. That is family-centered care, and it can be done on a constant basis."

"I'm a believer," I said.

"Compassion and care should go hand-in-hand," Barb said in way of summary.

"Thank you for taking time to share your ideas with me," I said.

Barb got up and moved away from the table. We headed out of the cafeteria and down the hall to the bank of elevators. As we said good-bye, out of the corner of my eye, I noticed the two most outstanding reasons for the ideas behind family-centered care. There, in full glory, were the two young boys who I'd seen on the way in. The mother adjusted the red ski cap on one of the boys. As she headed to the same door through which I was leaving, she took their mitten-covered hands and led them back into the world.

Family-centered care? Barb was absolutely right. It isn't just an idea; it is the only way to practice health care.

CHAPTER 15

The Story of Olivia Stockmeyer
Part IV

"Miracles occur naturally as expressions of love.
The real miracle is the love that inspires them.
In this sense everything that comes from love is a miracle."
—*Marianne Williamson*

There was little doubt that Kevin and Kim Stockmeyer felt as if they were caught in the trap of a deep nightmare. Dr. Budi had just explained that it might be necessary to place Olivia on the ECMO machine that would support her life. "It was a pretty routine surgery, or so we believed," Kim said. "And Olivia was pretty close to death. We were simply out of our minds with grief. Kevin and I were in a complete state of shock."

"Yet, there's that voice in the back of your head that tells you to be strong," Kevin said. "Honestly, thinking back on it, I'm not sure how we got through that very moment."

"Chaplain Betty," Kim said. "She was right there beside us. Chaplain Betty kept us together when all we wanted to do was fall apart."

Kim, Kevin, and Kim's father carefully approached the bed with Chaplain Betty by their side. "We knew that Olivia's oxygen saturation had to improve drastically, but we also understood that it was a long shot given all that she'd been through that afternoon," Kim said. "I felt almost ridiculous, but we circled the bed and began to pray. We held hands and said the 'Our Father' and a 'Hail Mary' as we cried."

"It gives me the chills to think of it," Kevin said, "but as we prayed, I kept my eyes glued to the monitors and I noticed that Olivia's oxygen saturation and heart rate were improving. They improved enough, in that short span of time, that she did not need the ECMO machine."

As Kim listened to Kevin explain what happened, her eyes filled with tears. "I don't know where we'd be without Chaplain Betty," she whispered. "At that moment, I felt as though God had sent Chaplain Betty to be with us. It was just so miraculous to us. We were in complete disbelief that Olivia had improved in the time that we were praying."

Olivia was placed in a medically-induced coma in an effort to allow for healing. "We were still so scared," Kim said. "We certainly leaned on the hospital support group and our family for guidance"

Kevin and Kim's family was right there for support. After staying with Olivia in the room for a short while, the couple returned to the waiting room. Much to their appreciation, their extended family had gathered in support of Olivia. "Our support system was just unbelievable," Kevin said. "Family members came on a moment's notice to be with us. Some of them traveled from as far away as Franklinville and Lockport. We can never truly thank them enough. When we needed them there, they came."

That night, Kim stayed beside Olivia. Complete and utter exhaustion took hold of Kim's body, but she held her daughter's hand, and whispered words of love. "She needed to know I was there."

The emergency was over, but the healing process would be quite lengthy. On that Sunday night, Olivia needed a blood transfusion because her blood was not carrying enough oxygen. Olivia was on a sedative and a paralytic to keep her from moving so that she wouldn't fight the ventilator that she so desperately needed.

"Olivia's nurse that night was Kathy Humphrey," Kim said. "Kathy didn't stop working all night. She was so calm and comforting, and so unbelievably efficient. Just watching her work was amazing, and I thank God that she was there for Olivia that night."

As the Stockmeyers recount the horror of the emergency in the PICU, they are quick to mention the care and compassion of the staff. They are also extremely hesitant to assess blame. The questions in their minds remained, but as the shock wore off, they found that their determination soared. Olivia would be just fine, but she had to be, because as a family, the Stockmeyers believed that there was no alternative. Yet that's not to say that they weren't scared out of their minds as the emergency of March 6, 2005 extended to the morning of March 7, 2005.

* * *

The emergency of the previous day hung over every move that the Stockmeyers made on Monday, March 7th. The parents of a very sick child involved in an acute emergency situation are often suspended in a state of disbelief that is tempered with complete and utter exhaustion. Parents often times feel a tremendous sense of loss as they understand that they are extremely unprepared to care for their sick child. For Kevin and Kim, this realization was absolutely heartbreaking. "It's a tough pill to swallow," Kim explained. "From the moment when Olivia took her first breath, we were there for her. Our job is to protect her and care for her, and make sure that all of her needs are met. When Olivia's condition worsened on Sunday, we understood that we were no longer in control of what happened to her. It didn't really matter that we loved her so much. It didn't matter that we didn't want her to be sick. We were at the mercy of the situation and the feeling that you aren't in control of your child's well-being is heartbreaking."

Yet the Stockmeyers worked hard to gain back some semblance of control. "We asked a lot of questions, and we tried hard to understand what had happened, and what was necessary for Olivia to make a full recovery," Kevin said. "Kim started to keep a diary of what was happening. We took an active role in Olivia's treatment, and we tried to prepare ourselves as best as we could."

The anxiety in such a situation also manifests itself in a number of different ways. "There's a great deal of trust that must be extended to the people who are caring for your child," Kevin said. "Just a day before, or a couple of days before, the doctors and nurses were not a part of our life. We were meeting these people at a very crucial time. We were placing our trust in them to take care of our child when she was facing the most difficult of battles. There is doubt involved because, as a parent, you want your sick child in the hands of the very best and most capable men and women. Of course, as you're going through it, you don't understand all of what is happening, but God, you are really hoping that their instincts are true. It certainly crossed our minds that we wanted the best of all care for Olivia. Not knowing a lot about the hospital, we wondered if she was in the right place."

Kim's notes in her diary were a detailed description of treatment as described by the hospital staff:

03/07/05—Increased mean airway pressure of ventilator from 22 to 23 in order to resolve the fluid build-up in the lungs. The fluid build-up is expected at this stage due to the body's reaction. On the ventilator the pressure only goes into the lungs and not everywhere as with the Bi-Pap machine. Urine is getting lighter.

As the reality of what was happening took hold, the Stockmeyers began to understand that Olivia's recovery would take quite a bit of time. "The little things that you worried about just a few days before are a hundred million miles away," Kevin said. "We were asking each other a lot of questions about vacation time and personal days. We were prepared to do whatever we needed to do to be there with Olivia. We tried hard to gain control of the things we could control."

"The very worst part of it is the doubt," Kim said. "While I was facing forward and trying hard to stay positive, there was that nagging thought in the back of my mind: What if she wasn't all right? How could we possibly handle that?"

The Stockmeyers slowly learned to trust those who were in charge of Olivia's care. Kim's notes on Olivia's progress contained the names of those who were charged with the task of ensuring that Olivia was getting the best of treatment:

03/08/05—7:49 a.m—Nurse Heidi—Very good night. Don't have the result of the culture test yet. The goal is to reduce nitric oxide to zero and transfer Olivia to a regular respirator in order for her to be portable to do a CT-scan. The CT-scan is necessary due to the loss of oxygen on the 6th (routine). After Olivia is more stable they will run tests to see how the pulmonary edema occurred in the first place.

Years later, the Stockmeyers would sacrifice their time to assist other families in similar situations. Both Kim and Kevin are extremely giving of their time as they consider the care that Olivia received. "It is important that the parents and the staff members work together," Kim said. "I'm not sure how well we would have been able to handle it if we were left in the dark about the details of Olivia's recovery. We wanted to be treated with respect. It's funny because neither Kevin nor myself had any sort of medical background, and we were hearing some words for the very first time. Parents belong in the loop as far as the care of their child is concerned. We wanted to know why Olivia was going for a CT-Scan. We wanted to know how long she would be on a ventilator and why she was receiving the medicine that was being administered. The staff members that we were working with were very responsive to our questions. They comforted us, made information and services available to us, and offered guidance. I can't even begin to think what it might have been like if they weren't cooperative."

While Olivia had survived the emergency of March 6, two days later Kim and Kevin were still on pins and needles. "There's a certain part of you that wants to scream out," Kevin said. "It's almost like you want to yell, 'Enough is enough'. In the meantime, you're worried about everything else. I was worried about Kim and how she was holding up, and she was worried about me. It's easy to forget that you're in it together, because as a person you have your own fears and misconceptions, but we did pretty well. Again, the rest of our family stepped up to the plate and helped us through it."

Kim's notes are tempered with caution. Her second entry for March 8th speaks of her concerns. *03/08/05—2 p.m.—Took chest X-ray. Looks better than yesterday. One lung is clear - the other is still 'sick', cloudy. Will wait longer to change respirator. As of 7:50 p.m. nitric oxide is down to 1. Plan to give hemoglobin tonight.*

As Olivia's treatment continued, the Stockmeyers were exposed to the highs and the lows of having a very sick child. The blood cultures, urine cultures and tracheal aspirate cultures were negative for WBC or organisms. Yet, on March 12th, Olivia tested positive for RSV, a respiratory virus.

"So much happened during that first week of Olivia's recovery," Kim explained. The chest X-rays would just show the secretions moving around. Olivia's lung collapsed on one occasion, but quickly reinflated. The hole in the lung hadn't repaired itself, and we learned to keep an eye on all of her stats to make sure that she didn't need suction. I never thought I'd be worried about nitrous oxide levels, or when or why she needed hemoglobin, but that's where we were. When Olivia tested positive for RSV, we were fairly devastated, because it simply meant that her recovery time was going to be much, much longer."

03/12/05—Last night tested positive for RSV. Moved into isolation room. Chest X-ray looked better than morning. Suctioned and removed a lot of secretions - secretions coming out of nose. This morning's X-ray showed that her left lung was clearer than yesterday. Upper right lung hazier than yesterday. Plan today is to stay the course.

Of course, Kim and Kevin had no idea if the hole in Olivia's lung would heal. There are few guarantees when it comes to the treatment of a sick child. Given the fact that Olivia's cleft palate surgery was usually a fairly routine surgery, and that she was now fighting for her life, the parents weren't taking anything for granted.

"The things that go through your head are pretty devastating," Kevin said. "Given our support system we were able to balance our routine when Olivia was in the PICU, but there are those scary moments when you're alone with your thoughts. No matter how positive everyone is in the treatment, there comes a moment when you realize that it is your baby there under the covers, and that her very life hangs in the balance."

Kim continued to take notes and the hospital staff continually tested Olivia to ensure that all of the bases were covered. "The care received in the PICU was simply amazing," Kim said. "The doctors and nurses were so attentive, and it seemed as though they were prepared for every new possible symptom. Looking back, their diligence is almost too much to comprehend. We are certainly appreciative of the efforts of everyone involved in Olivia's care."

Still, the trip out of the woods was a long one.

"I can remember one day when I was really down," Kim said. "The resident, Omar S. Al-Ibrahim, noticed that I was having a difficult time of it and he flat-out told me, 'You need to be very strong for Olivia today.' As simple as that statement was, it made me focus on the task at hand, and Olivia had a good day."

03/13/05—Having a very good day, chest X-ray from this morning was improved from yesterday. Urinating very frequently and that is a good sign that she is moving fluids. They are going to try to start removing chest tubes one at a time over the next several days. 100% O_2 saturation, reducing O_2 level. On X-ray there is a faint line on the lower right lung. May be the division between the upper and lower lobes. Took chest tube out of suction. If no bubbles are seen, will remove chest tube."

Perhaps the very worst of days was the stretch between March 16, and March 17 when one of Kim and Kevin's potential worries surfaced. Both Kim and Kevin made entries into the daily diary that was now a staple of communication in Olivia's care.

03/16/05—Had a bad night—high CO_2. Tried to turn prone, that made her worse. Turned back. Last night, X-ray showed that she had 2 pockets of air—one in upper and lower right lung. This morning, back to normal. Good sign that her body handled the overnight changes well. Plan is to wean off pressure on ventilator, down to 23 at 11:00. Morning X-ray was good—little pocket of air in lower right lung.

03/17/05—Overnight her CO_2 was rising and her pupils were different sizes. When pupils are different sizes it could mean that something is happening in the brain. Did a CT-scan of the head and chest—came *back normal. Will do an EEG to test brain wave activity to make sure there were no seizures. Pupil reaction could be a result of elevated CO_2. Switched to regulator ventilator and she is tolerating that well! CT-scan showed that her brain is a little small and the space around (fluid) her brain is a little larger. Nothing of concern now, watch developmentally.*

Kim and Kevin spoke as one as they considered the time that Olivia struggled in the PICU. The days seemed much longer somehow and the young parents were introduced to elevated concepts of faith, hope, and trust. Together, they worked their way through, but fighting even harder than them was Olivia.

"She fought so hard," Kim said with tears blasting their way to the front of her eyes. "It was so hard to see her like that. The crying and the discomfort ate a hole through our hearts. We felt so helpless, you know? There was a point in her treatment when Olivia couldn't maintain her oxygen level and she was placed under an oxygen tent. That was so hard for me because I couldn't touch her face. I can clearly remember how upset that made me. I just wanted to touch my daughter, and comfort her. We were worried about respiratory distress and drug withdrawal, and a hundred-and-one different things."

"And being in the hospital, day after day and night after night just wears you down," Kevin said. "It was so unreal to be traveling back and forth while the rest of life was going on all around us. It's not like you care what is happening in the outside world, but deep down, you understand that the rest of the world is going on without you. It's a lonely feeling, and we certainly sympathize with the parents of children who will never be well. That would be too much to handle."

Of course, as Olivia's condition very slowly improved, Kim and Kevin's hopes soared. The moment that the family had been anticipating finally came on March 22nd at 6:45 a.m.

"We were so excited that Olivia was being taken off the ventilator," Kim said. "To us it was a real sign that she was going to make it through the whole ordeal, but more than anything else, we wanted our vibrant, happy child back. We had missed her so much."

The anticipated moment did not work out very well. "The first day that she came off of the ventilator was actually one of the worst days," Kevin said.

"Olivia was going through major drug withdrawal," Kim explained. "We were waiting for a healthy child, but Olivia wasn't the child we knew. All she could do was moan, and the idea that she was suffering from drug withdrawal, at fourteen months, was almost too much to handle."

Kim and Kevin can barely stand to think of that day and how much it hurt all of those around Olivia. "My mom was so excited that day," Kim said. "When all that Olivia could do was moan, Mom was just so upset. I get a sick feeling in the pit of my stomach when I think back to that day, because not only was Olivia not quite back yet, but Mom was hurting too. We all felt pretty helpless."

Despite the ups and downs of the treatment plan, there was one single moment that stood out for the parents.

"I was way down in the dumps," Kim said. "I'm not sure what was happening with Olivia at the moment, but I must have showed some real signs of stress because Dr. Hernan said the words that I had longed to hear. "This isn't a child that is dying. This is a child that is sick and getting well."

It was all that the Stockmeyers needed to hear to find the strength to make it through the rest of Olivia's stay.

CHAPTER 16

The Story of Anthony Stinson
Part IV

*"Most of the important things in the world
have been accomplished by people who have kept trying when
there seemed to be no hope at all."*
—Dale Carnegie

Very often, when faced with insurmountable tasks, the easiest thing to do is to complain about the hand you are dealt. In every walk of life there are people who are more comfortable stuck in a state of constant negativity. People find it easy to complain when their coffee is too hot or too cold. They complain when there isn't anything suitable to watch on television, or if the sports team they're rooting for doesn't win. They complain as they wake in the morning that the weather is just plain terrible, and they go to bed at night complaining that the weather tomorrow isn't going to be any better.

As the Stinson family prepared for Anthony's return home from the hospital after a four-month stay, there was precious little time to complain about anything.

"I was deathly afraid of coming home," Trina explained. "I didn't have much of an idea about how I was going to be able to care for Anthony. There was so much that I needed to learn, and his illness left him so damaged that I never thought I'd be able to cope."

Four years later, as I scanned the living area I was unbelievably impressed by the job that Trina had done. While Anthony's
crib in the center of the room would be a horrible inconvenience
to anyone prone to complain about their plight in life, Trina had
made the house a very comfortable home for both of her
children.

"I remember those first few days so well. I spent every
moment by Anthony's side. I either sat in the chair beside his bed
or fell asleep on the floor at the foot of the bed. I was so afraid of
not being by him if something were to happen." Trina's voice fell
off and she came as close to complaining as she possibly can. "Life
has been very difficult," she said. "When we brought him home
from the hospital, I was petrified to even administer his medicines. Anthony would have seizures all day, and he would cry and
cry. I tried to do everything I could to soothe him. Anthony was
just thirty-five pounds in those days, so I could hold him and
rock him, but nothing seemed to work. I would sing to him and
give him Tylenol or Motrin, but he was just so uncomfortable.
Do you know how difficult it is for a mother not to be able to
soothe her child?"

Trina turned to her son. Anthony was no longer thirty-five
pounds. He was approximately eighty pounds, and it was difficult
for Trina to hold him these days.

"Now, when he needs to be comforted I lie beside him, letting my head touch his head. I sing to him and just touch him to
let him know that I'm still here."

As unbelievably efficient as Trina is now, the homecare of
Anthony did not come easy.

"I learned Anthony's care through a lot of trial and error. His
case is extremely complex, and it's impossible to find the answers
in a medical book. It literally took years to figure out what worked
for him. It's funny because, if you asked me what I did over the
weekend, I would have to think about it, but if you ask me anything about Anthony, I could recite everything from the day he
was born to today."

"So, I see the list of medications and the chalkboard assignments of care, but tell me about some of the things you worry about on a daily basis," I said.

"First of all, it's the 'mom' in me that knows what he needs daily. For instance, I know that he cannot lie in the same position for more than two hours because of a possible skin breakdown. I have to make sure I remember when his last bowel movement was, and if he needs assistance. I have to consider whether or not to call GI to get him on a different regime because this one doesn't work anymore. I have to evaluate whether he's having more seizures today, and if I should call neurology, or wait a little longer to see if they subside. I need to assess if his lungs can clear with his vest, or a cough assist, or suctioning, or do I need to call the lung center?"

Trina offered a sheepish smile as I lowered my pen and stared at her in disbelief.

"He rarely gets fevers because of the temperature control in his brain, so if his temperature is elevated, I have to figure out if he has an infection. Does he need an antibiotic? Does he need extra oxygen? Does he need blood drawn to see if any bacteria grows? Trach culture? Step up on his vest, cough assist and chest PT?"

Trina was clicking off a list in her mind. I sensed that each thing she was speaking to me about was on a running list that starts over with each new day.

"His shoulders and hips are slightly dislocated, so I need to make sure that all new nurses and therapists do his range of motion and reposition him so they don't hurt him. If he's sleeping all the time, I need to get a script from neuro and take him to WCHOB to get his ammonia level tested. If it's elevated, we need to decrease depakene or increase carnitor, or both."

"And how did you learn all of this? I know that being a mom is your inspiration, but you've basically passed one medical course after another."

"I will learn all I need to learn," Trina said. "Sarah Johnson was Anthony's first homecare nurse, and I honestly don't know where I'd be without Sarah. She showed me how to take care of Anthony. It took so much time to get him on a strict respiratory schedule and to balance his medications so that they were spread apart equally. Sarah went to the doctor appointments with me, and because of her medical backgrounds she was able to discern what the doctors were telling me. Sarah would break it all down for me so that I understood. Together we were able to establish a plan to make Anthony as comfortable as possible."

Despite Sarah's invaluable help, the climb often seemed too steep for Trina to handle.

"I hated the fact that there were strangers coming to my home to help. Even now, I must trust the nurse who comes in. If I don't, they leave. At the beginning, though, it was hard. All the while I was wishing that I had my own life back, I was learning that if Anthony wasn't seizing all the time, he was in respiratory distress or vomiting and at an increased risk of contracting aspiration pneumonia. Just when I would become educated and used to one particular issue, something else would start."

These days Trina speaks like a seasoned veteran of the medical community. "Long ago I committed to the care of my son. During those first few days, I promised myself that no matter what happened, I would be there for him. Come hell or high water, Anthony knows I am right here beside him."

Trina's words went straight to my heart, but I brushed aside my own feelings and listened to the determined voice of a wonderful mother.

"There was so much to balance and figure out. There were certainly moments when I felt as if we were completely abandoned by the medical community. It was so difficult to balance Anthony's medications and figure out the proper therapies. I spent a lot of time fighting for nursing care and dealing with insurance denials. I had to learn the best way to transport Anthony to the emergency room or to his doctor appointments. Anthony's health was so poor that I also realized that at any moment there could be an emergency that could take him from me forever. Realizing that hurt me more than anything else."

Yet Trina's resolve proved to be stronger than the undiagnosed illness that had forever trapped her son. "I gathered every single piece of information about Anthony from the very first moment of his life to the exact moment when I began sending out inquiries, contacting doctors all over the country in an effort to find an answer or a cure."

Trina's voice faded to a whisper. "I tried to think of everything. I figured that even the tiniest detail might make a difference to a doctor who was reading the case for the first time. I was desperate for help. Compiling the information to send out and taking care of Anthony full-time left me very little time to grieve. I suppose that I truly didn't want to. Through all of it, I tried real hard to let Nicholas know that I still loved him as much as his brother. Anthony had so much of my attention that I did my best to show Nicholas that I was still there for him too. I volunteered weekly at his school. I attended as many school functions as I could, and I did my best to make Nicholas feel special. I arranged for a counselor to come to the home to speak with Nicholas about how to express some of the things that might be confusing him about Anthony's illness."

My mind shifted to the moment when I first encountered Nicholas at the front door. He had been accepting of me from the very first moment. He was polite, enthusiastic, and so full of life. I thought of the adjustments that he had to make as I considered his mother's words.

"At first, I told Nick that Anthony would get better. I honestly believed it too, but as time went on and Anthony just got sicker and required more support to keep him alive and comfortable, I had to come face-to-face with the fact that this was how my boy was going to be for the rest of his life. Nicholas' counselor asked me if I ever cried in front of him. Of course, I hadn't let him see me cry! But the counselor told me that it was okay to cry in front of Nicholas. I think that it was at that point that we started to heal a little bit."

Trina bowed her head and took a deep breath. I couldn't imagine how she was keeping it together enough not to cry in front of me because I was on the verge of tears myself.

"I told Nick that Anthony would get better some day because

I really wanted to shield him from the pain. The counselor explained it for me by saying something that I live by to this day. She explained that I should not try to protect my children from pain, loss, or change, but that I should give them the tools to cope with the difficult things that life would throw their way."

Trina's ability to cope with difficult situations was severely tested. It was certainly a test that many others could easily fail.

"I don't give up easily," Trina explained. "Anthony's quality of life was pretty poor. More than anything else, I wanted to make him more comfortable. I suppose that every mother wants that for her child, right? I called doctor after doctor to see if there was some sort of test they could do to balance everything so that Anthony wasn't in so much distress. When it was explained to me that I had done all that I could, I was deeply offended. I felt that the harder I tried, the worse the situation became. It is a difficult situation because I need to write letters to justify almost everything that Anthony requires. Although, at this point, I know more about Anthony's required care than anyone, because the insurance company doesn't see MD after my name, I need to send the information to the appropriate doctor, who then sends a letter back to me, that I forward to the insurance company. Everything is a major pain, but I do it because I won't give up."

Giving up was never actually an option that Trina would even consider. The more uncomfortable Anthony was, the more determined his mother became.

"Doctors and nurses approached me about the idea of 'Do Not Resuscitate Orders'. I just wanted to scream. I never would wish anyone the excruciating pain that I was feeling, but I wondered if they would consider DNR if it were their child lying in that bed."

Trina was quick to point out that, despite their insistence that everything possible had been done for Anthony, there wasn't a doctor who didn't respond to her requests.

"If I thought of a disease or wanted to see another doctor, or needed a letter written, there wasn't one doctor who wasn't willing to help me."

The first year of Anthony's homecare passed extremely slowly. The Stinsons were forced to deal with one emergency after another. Anthony was hospitalized on numerous occasions for any number of situations that could easily tear him from his mother's arms. Eventually, Anthony needed a tracheotomy because of the constant aspiration pneumonias that damaged his lungs so badly that one day he would require a ventilator.

"I haven't heard his voice since May 28, 2003," Trina explained. "When he got sick in April of 2002, he lost his ability to speak, but I could still hear him cry or make noises. The tracheotomy took even that away from me."

Of course, realizing how much she lost caused Trina to reflect on the bigger picture.

"When Anthony first got sick, I seriously doubted that there was a God. Why would God do such a thing to my son, or any other child in the world? What sort of God would put my son through such a thing? I clearly remember that when Anthony got sick some friends of ours put together a benefit for us. At the benefit, a woman I had never met before handed me a framed poem entitled "Anthony's Special Mother". I read the poem and I cried, but as time went on, my doubts about the existence of God continued to grow, and eventually, I put the poem in a drawer and forgot about it. How could there be a God?"

Trina didn't answer her own question right away. Instead, she thought back on the gradual decline of her beautiful son "When Nicholas was born, as a mother, I always felt that I could fix anything that was wrong. Mommies do that, right?" Trina's expressive eyes flashed a knowing glance as she forced a smile. "If Nicholas got an ear infection, I took him to the doctor and got antibiotics that would clear it up. If he skinned his knee, I would place a band-aid over the cut and kiss him and hold him until he felt better. I did the same thing with Anthony when he was young. Maybe I was too close to the situation, but I didn't notice the slow decline of Anthony. I was so busy making him feel comfortable that I couldn't recognize how much he had degenerated. I think about that every single day. I knew that there was something more wrong with Anthony when his blindness and unbalance presented themselves, but the doctors couldn't pinpoint it so we adapted."

No matter how hard she tried, Trina would never be able to shake the memory of April 19, 2002.

"How could I believe that there was a God? When he woke up from that medically induced coma, and all of his abilities had been stripped, I was as sick as I could possibly be. I couldn't just kiss him and make it better. I still try and hold him hard enough to make his pain go away, but it'll never really work the way that I want it to work."

Every time that it appeared that Trina was on the verge of giving into her pain, she reached deep into her reservoir of strength.

"When people who have never met Anthony look at him, they feel as if the only thing he can do is look off into space, but when you get to know him now, you can still see the boy that is trapped somewhere deep inside. When he is having a 'good' day, he'll smile at me. Sometimes he'll use his eyes to respond to yes and no questions."

Trina allowed me a glimpse into how she regained her trust in God and the faith and strength that she summons on a daily basis in an attempt to cope.

"Sometimes it'll be months before he smiles again, but when he does, my heart threatens to explode. I get tears in my eyes because I know my boy is still with me. I know that he knows that I love him, and I thank God because He allows me a bright moment."

Trina Stinson did not allow herself time to complain.

CHAPTER 17

The Story of Dr. Doron Feldman

*"Achievement seems to be connected with action.
Successful men and women keep moving.
They make mistakes but they don't quit."*
—*Conrad Hilton*

More than half a world away, Uri Feldman is the accomplished leader of the Dielectric Spectroscopy Laboratory at the Hebrew University of Jerusalem. Uri Feldman is an extremely prolific scientist and author whose theories are well-received and well-respected throughout the world. Uri Feldman has established a body of work that grants him a legacy of good will and ambition that will stretch across lifetimes. If there is one simple thing that his son, Doron Feldman, the Chief of Anesthesiology at The Women & Children's Hospital of Buffalo, wants it is to follow in his father's footsteps. More than anything else, Doron Feldman, clearly sees the bigger picture, and he fully understands that his work is important to families, as well as to his co-workers. I met with Doron on a Saturday afternoon in his office at The Women & Children's Hospital of Buffalo. Doron was in full scrubs, with a mask hanging around his neck. He had just completed his work in an operation that had gone well. We sat across from one another and talked about everything from the Iraq war to our mutual love of dogs. As I worked on the story of Dr. Doron Feldman, it occurred to me that I was meeting with a man who was well on his way to establishing a legacy that would make both his parents and his children proud. I began the interview with the question that I had asked each of his co-workers.

"How do you handle the endless parade of sick children?"

"The real challenge is keeping everything in perspective," Doron said. "I have three healthy children, and being here each and every day allows me the chance to see that I am very blessed. Of course, another way of looking at it is to understand that there are two million people in our catchment area, and it sort of works like a funnel because we wind up seeing all of the misery. I try and tell myself that there are a lot of healthy children out there living extremely normal lives."

"Does seeing the misery change the way you raise your children?"

"I'm cautious and fearful for my children's safety. Even more so than my wife, I would imagine, because I see some difficult things on a daily basis. There are a lot of cases that grab you, and I truly hurt for some of these kids. Off the top of my head, I think of a child who was badly injured in an ATV accident and is in a vegetative state. My heart aches for that child and his family. I think of a sixteen-year-old who was unrestrained in a car accident and is completely paralyzed from the neck down. He was a child that I spoke with before the operation, and he asked me if he would be able to perform a simple task that he had performed very well. I almost broke down when he asked the question."

"Exactly," I said. "That has to be a difficult thing to face."

"Certainly it is," Dr. Feldman said. "Yet the high point of doing this work is meeting a child who is very sick, who we can make well. I often think of your own son when I consider our work. His case was a perfect example of how rewarding this job could be."

I squirmed in my chair, but nodded along. Dr. Feldman had been in the operating room with Jake. By all accounts, it was the expert work of Dr. Feldman that had been crucial to my son's survival in the removal of the tumor.

"The difficult part is when we work with children who are suffering with chronic diseases that can't be easily handled. My heart is truly aching right now because there's a young man in here now who recently suffered a stroke. A young boy who has a stroke for no apparent reason is difficult to process."

"As an anesthesiologist, you probably don't have quite the one-on-one contact that the patient's doctor or the surgeon might have, correct?"

"That's right, we don't deal with the family to that extent, but I go into each operation knowing that if I were to make a mistake and deprive the patient of oxygen to the brain or heart, the quality of the patient's life could be damaged for the next 80 years. It's different dealing with children because the span of life is greater. Overall, being prepared is the key."

"In a number of conversations that I've had for this story, God plays a prominent role in how healthcare professionals are able to balance some of the misery."

"Absolutely," Dr. Feldman said. "Yet the random, brutal, unexplainable can certainly shake the foundation of your faith. I certainly believe in God, but you wonder sometimes about the notion of an all-loving or all-powerful God. It might very well be a different sort of God."

"But you enjoy your job," I said.

"I love my job. I am extremely lucky to be given the opportunity to practice medicine. It's a tough job; we work nights, weekends, and holidays. The hours are long; we are always under the cloud of being sued for just doing our work."

"I was going to ask you about that," I said.

"It's horrendous," Dr. Feldman said. "The threat of litigation is destroying the trust that is intrinsic in the doctor-patient relationship, but there isn't a lot of time to worry about it. As a physician you are defensive about it because you hear the stories, but I can't get emotionally wrapped up in it because there's too much to do. The best way to handle it is to be meticulous, personable and conscientious. What else is there?"

"How about angry patients or family members? How do you cope with that in your working environment?"

"I understand that people are in the most stressful of all situations. If there is anger, I accept it. I don't take it personally because I know that it's not me they're angry with; they are angry with their circumstances right at that moment."

"So, we handled a couple of the difficult aspects of your job right off the bat. Tell me why you love this job."

"That's easy," Dr. Feldman said with a smile. "We are afforded tremendous respect, we have a wonderful working environment, and there are a lot of days when I can look back at my work and realize that what I did mattered. You know, I learned that from my father. My dad, Uri, is a tough, knowledgeable man. He's an extremely prolific writer, has his Ph.D. in physics and is extremely well-respected in his field of study. I speak with him almost every day, and his opinion truly matters to me. His life is a great example to me, and I respect him to the ends of the earth for what he's been able to accomplish."

"And your mom?"

"Dalia, my mom, is the best possible mom that you can imagine. She was the glue that held everything together, and she allowed my father to pursue his goals. Together they raised three boys. My brother Tomer is an ER physician in Virginia, and my brother Ronen is a computer engineer. We're all doing well, and that is a testament to the legacy that my parents built together."

"You've mentioned legacy and a bigger picture. What about your legacy?"

"I've been with my wife, Deborah, for twenty-five years, and we've been married for twenty. We have three children, Leeshi, who is a sophomore at The University at Buffalo, Daniel, who just made his JV-Hockey Team—so he's an extremely proud young man right about now—and Jacob, who is thirteen and is just a great and wonderful boy. I am very close to my children and my family is my world."

"I would imagine that the long hours would be something that would make you cherish your time with the kids even more."

"Exactly. I'm on call today so I'm here for a 24-hour stretch. I can reasonably expect a 70 to 80 hour workweek, and it is difficult. It ages you. There aren't a lot of days when the pager isn't going off, but I try and handle things as they come. I like to be prepared, and that is the best way to handle this work."

"What about relaxation? Golf?"

"No, golf, as Mark Twain said, is a good walk spoiled," Dr. Feldman said with a laugh. "There are difficult aspects to this job, and perhaps one of them is finding the time to do the things that you love to do."

"I suppose that another difficult aspect of your job is treating victims of child abuse."

Dr. Feldman's face quickly changed expression as a pained look took control. "The hospital has an excellent system for reporting abuse cases and contacting social services, but just the idea of it infuriates me. It is simply cruelty for cruelty's sake, and it makes me question my beliefs. There isn't much more to say about it, really. The perpetrators have to be punished to the fullest extent of the law."

Dr. Feldman shrugged because there is precious little else to say about the subject. The heavy, almost desperate feeling in the room is something that we are both uncomfortable with.

"Tell me about how it feels to work at this hospital. Are you proud to be here?"

"Unbelievably proud," Dr. Feldman answered. "There have been tremendous improvements made over the past four or five years, and while we've always had very talented doctors on staff, now we are working with excellent equipment. The feeling is extremely positive, and we have a good administrative staff in place. The administration is very approachable and open to change. The Chief Medical Officer is Dr. James Foster, a very bright, practical, forward-thinking man who listens to and works with the staff. I am extremely proud of the efforts of everyone associated with this hospital."

"And yet, there are difficulties. The emergency room is often crowded and takes some time to navigate."

"Absolutely," Dr. Feldman said. "Yet you have to remember that this is an institution where we help everyone, regardless of circumstance. Perhaps there are things that can be done differently, but on a grand scale, I'm proud of the fact that we take care of people. That is the bottom line."

"You work with hundreds of people. I'm sure that there are people who do not live up to your high standards in every instance."

"That's human nature," Dr. Feldman replied with a shrug. "Certainly there are people who do not behave in a professional manner, but that is true everywhere. As the head of a department, you have to try and marginalize those people and the instances where this occurs. It's difficult to work with practitioners who proclaim that they don't work nights and weekends, but you adjust and you learn to count on those who share your passion."

"You have a lot of athletes who come into the hospital and draw tremendous amounts of attention. Does it seem a little unbalanced to you that you work to save children, but that you don't receive a portion of the attention that someone who plays a game receives?"

"I don't have a problem with any of it," Dr. Feldman answered. "I appreciate the fact that the athletes stop by and pay attention to the children. As individuals, I don't know of one staff member who is looking for attention, and I don't think that anyone's job is more important than anyone else's. In my eyes, the guy who drives the bus that delivers my children to school has a very important job. He's responsible for the safety of 40 children. I'm only really working with one at a time."

"So, this is where you want to be at this stage of your career," I said.

"I had a nightmare a few years ago," Dr. Feldman murmured. "I dreamed that I wasn't working here, and let me tell you, I woke up in a cold sweat. In this business, there are always offers to move to other institutions. The grass isn't greener elsewhere. I love Buffalo and the work we are doing here."

"Tell me about the Department of Anesthesiology."

"We have a 24/7 in-house staff made up of residents, fellows, nurse anesthesiologists, and attending physicians. We all work together and take turns being on call. I think it is extremely important that I am willing to do anything that I am asking others to do. The departmental goal is to always be prepared and to take responsibility for our actions. As I tell my residents, I would rather be afraid because I know what can happen than be afraid because I am clueless. Being properly prepared takes a lot of the unnecessary fear out of a given situation."

"So if you had a motto to go by, what would it be?"

"Your lack of planning does not constitute an emergency on my part," Dr. Feldman said with a laugh. "Seriously, in this line of work, being prepared is a major part of the battle."

"I imagine that your sense of discipline shows itself in other aspects of your life. What sort of hobbies do you have?"

"My kids are my main hobby, of course, but I'm also an avid gun collector, I enjoy target shooting, and I do quite a bit of reading. I enjoy biographies, and American and Russian military histories. Since I travel quiet a bit, I download books on tape to my I-pod and I'll listen to them that way."

Dr. Feldman's confession that he owned an I-pod triggered another question. "I recently read *The Making of a Surgeon*," I said. "It was a wonderful story written by Dr. William A. Nolen, but it was written over 30 years ago, and I found that the medicine seemed primitive in those days compared to what is available today. Do you find it disconcerting that there are people in this country who can't afford healthcare?"

"There are liars, damn liars and statisticians. It all depends upon how you look at it," Dr. Feldman answered. "Think about all of the advancements in medicine since the time when Dr. Nolen wrote that book. The costs have been astronomical, right? It's difficult to offer 2007 healthcare at 1975 prices. Besides, what part does not having healthcare play here? We will treat all-comers. Excellent healthcare is available. America is the greatest country in the history of mankind. Sometimes people complain without thinking about all sides of an issue, but the situation isn't quite as dire as some people make it out to be."

We are approaching the end of the interview, but there is one huge question waiting patiently in the back of my mind. I am struggling with whether or not I want to hear the answer, but I am also well aware that Dr. Feldman's work was instrumental in the success of my son's operation. At the time, surgeon Marc Levitt had explained to me that the anesthesiologist would play a huge role. I decided to dance around the question of Jake's care and approached the subject carefully.

"Prior to every operation you'll hear that there is a risk anytime anyone is put under. Is that true of every operation?"

"Sure, there are risks," Dr. Feldman answered. "Of course, the goal is to minimize the potential for mistakes. A bad outcome is usually the result of a series of mistakes being made. By being prepared, the potential for such mistakes is greatly reduced."

I sighed heavily as I asked the question. "Do you remember my son's operation?"

"Of course, all the details," Dr. Feldman answered. "You want to hear about it?"

"I think," I answered. We both laughed.

Dr. Feldman's entire demeanor changed as he searched his mind for the details of Jake's operation. "It was November 5, 2001, right?"

"You remember the date?"

Dr. Feldman shrugged. "I remember that it was very important to see the X-ray. I also remember meeting with Dr. Levitt and Dr. Caty to discuss the case in detail. We were extremely cautious about doing the operation because of the position of the tumor. We understood that we needed to be very well prepared in order to be successful. I examined your son, I studied the charts, and I communicated with the others who were going to be in the operating room."

"What concerned you the most?" I asked.

"We had to be sure that we put him under properly, and then the position of the breathing tube promised to be tricky. It was all about the proper positioning of your son for the operation. The muscle tension in your son's chest was what was holding the tumor off of his heart. It stood to reason that when his muscles were relaxed, the tumor could put pressure on his heart, and that wouldn't have worked out too well."

As Dr. Feldman explained this to me, the air in the room seemed to have gone stale. I felt a wave of heat rushing through my body as I imagined my son on that operating room table.

"Your son went under really well, and the breathing tube was placed, and that went well also. We agreed that the best way to get it done was to position Jake in a sitting position and, although it was less convenient for the surgeons, it was what we needed to do."

My heart was firmly stuck in my throat. Dr. Feldman's expression was less clinical and more human than I possibly could have imagined. I could tell by his demeanor that Jake's case meant a great deal to him, but I'm not sure if it would have been any different if it were anyone else's child.

"Were you afraid?" I asked.

"Oh yeah," Dr. Feldman answered. "There were risks involved, so I was afraid for what might happen, but as I've explained, being afraid of what might happen is a whole different story than being afraid because you have no idea what could happen."

"For the record, as you were afraid, I was shitting my pants," I said.

Dr. Feldman laughed. "That's what I'm speaking of," he said. "The opportunity to work with children, in a truly team fashion, to make them healthy again, is the most rewarding job in the world."

Dr. Feldman was quick to acknowledge the work of Dr. Levitt and Dr. Caty, and the entire team of people who worked with Jake.

"Everyone that I've spoken with at the hospital does that," I remarked. "You all seem to defer a compliment by pointing out the work of others."

"That's because it's true," Dr. Feldman said. "Working at the hospital is a lot like getting through every other aspect of life. You have to work together, you have to be prepared, and you have to be open to suggestions. Each and every time I will try and do my job to the best of my abilities. I will never do anything that will jeopardize the health of a child, and I communicate with the people I'm working for and with. It's a philosophy that's worked well through the years."

Dr. Feldman's pager went off and I closed my notebook quickly as he made his way toward the telephone. As he spoke to whoever was on the other end of the line, I couldn't help but think about the father and son relationships that we had discussed. I thought of Uri Feldman and the influence that he's had on his son. I contemplated my own sons and the fact that Dr. Feldman understood all that I had to lose as he worked on my child. He had been afraid for what might happen, and he prepared himself to be ready for the unexpected. We had opened our discussion speaking of legacies and leaving something behind for the rest of the world. My son Jake was simply one case in an endless parade of sick children who are made well by the hands of men like Doron Feldman.

I didn't tell Dr. Feldman that I am proud of him. I didn't pretend to imply that his family must be extremely proud of what he does day in and day out. Instead, I waited as he concluded his telephone call, and then I simply extended my hand.

"Thank you," I said. They are just two simple words that carry the message of years and years of happiness for my entire family.

"It's always a pleasure to talk with you," Dr. Feldman answered.

As I escaped down the back stairs of the hospital to the cold drizzle of a miserable November day, I nearly broke into a song and dance. The world is certainly a better place because of men like Doron Feldman, and I understood that his is a legacy that would make any father proud.

CHAPTER 18

The Story of Olivia Stockmeyer
Part V

*"When God calls you to do something,
he enables you to do it."*
—*Robert Schuller*

These days the Stockmeyer household is alive with tension. It is not the sort of tension reserved for the medical emergencies spoken of in this story. Rather, it is the normal, wonderful tension created by having two young children. Kim and Kevin Stockmeyer are so thankful for the anxiety currently created by their children, Matthew, and of course, Olivia.

The very first interview I conducted for this book was completed at the Stockmeyer home. The very first person I met in regard to the interview was Olivia Stockmeyer. I wrote the initial words for this book with a photo of Olivia taped to my desktop. Knowing what I knew before I met her, it was impossible to chase the vision of Olivia's smile out of the front of my mind, but her photo was before me, just in case.

Kevin opened the door for me. Right there at his feet, was Olivia. She was talking a mile a minute already, asking me what I wanted, asking her dad why I was there, and showing me her stuff. Three steps into the door, I was introduced to her Barbie chair, told of her love for Dora the Explorer, and the movie, Monsters Inc.

"She loves to chat," Kevin said by way of introduction. We headed through the living room toward the kitchen. Kevin plucked a few of Olivia's toys from the carpet and he smiled as he did so. Kim moved through the house with Matthew in tow. I'm not sure if Kim was in the process of changing Matthew or simply feeding him. (Matthew was less than two months old when this interview was conducted.) I commented that I wasn't quite sure what my wife was doing when our babies were so young.

"I'm sorry," Kevin said. "We're trying to get things taken care of, but there are always distractions when the children are so young."

"I remember the days well," I said. "How's the sleep depravation?"

"I'll gladly take it," Kevin answered.

Our discussion took place in the kitchen of the Stockmeyer home. Kim and Kevin graciously set out a huge bowl of chips with nacho cheese sauce. Olivia's eyes locked onto the bowl, and she very clearly asked her father to set her up.

"She speaks very well," I said.

"It's amazing, isn't it?" Kevin replied.

"Given what she went through, it's astounding," I said.

"There was a time when we weren't certain that we'd ever get back to a life such as this," Kevin said.

Olivia dipped one of her chips in the cheese sauce. She took a huge bite, turned to me and smiled. I smiled back, but I failed to hold her attention. Despite the fact that she had plenty of cheese sauce, she asked her father for just a little more. Kevin happily filled her bowl.

"It's crazy around here," Kim said, as she sat at the table across from Olivia. The look of love was evident in Kim's eyes as she took in the sight of her daughter, who was now wearing a bit of the sauce on her face.

"It's a wonderful thing," I said.

"You've asked us what we learned from the experience," Kim said. "I guess the biggest lesson of all is that we have learned to smell the roses. We have busy professional lives. A lot of people do these days, and it is very easy to get caught up in the day-to-day business of what needs to be done. We've learned to take the time to appreciate what we have because it could change so quickly."

Kevin tended to Olivia's insistent dipping into the bowl and her pre-occupation with the bigger bowl that had even more of the cheese sauce. Still, he nodded along with his wife's assessment of what had been learned.

"It's funny because before Olivia was sick, I was caught up in the pursuit of a job promotion or a bonus, or impressing the boss," Kim explained. "After Olivia was born, we had the mind-set that the family would come first, but it's easy to get caught up in all of it."

"It's so easy to put in a little more time at work and believe that you can make up the difference on the weekends," Kevin said.

"We learned that it might not be possible to make up for lost time," Kim said. "After Olivia's hospital stay our priorities changed. What good would come of a new car, or more material things, if we lost time with our children? The most valuable thing that we have is our love for each other. We always knew that, but I guess you can say that we appreciate it a little more."

"We definitely learned to appreciate the fact that we have a roof over our heads, good jobs, and two healthy wonderful children," Kevin added. "It's easier than people think to forget their blessings."

"We also learned that we can't plan everything," Kim said. She seemed torn between the conversation and listening for Matthew, who was hopefully asleep upstairs.

"We are both people who like to plan for everything right down to the smallest of details, but we learned that planning for every eventuality just isn't practical," Kevin added.

"We had planned even the birth of the children," Kim said with a laugh. "Both Olivia and Matthew's births were scheduled C-sections. We even knew the sex of the children beforehand. Olivia's birth and surgery seriously threw our schedules for a loop."

"Since Olivia's surgery and recovery, we've learned to go with the flow a bit more," Kevin explained. He reached across the table and wiped a bit of the sauce away from Olivia's beautiful face. As he did so, Olivia looked at me once more. She let loose with a long, hurried dissertation about Dora the Explorer and I simply laughed.

"She talks fast," Kevin said. "You know, it's strange to say, but having a very sick child is almost a blessing in a way because it forces you to prioritize, appreciate life, and understand the role that you play as a parent. Even though Olivia was very young, we understand that our presence and support played a role in her recovery. She felt our anxieties, and she responded to us."

"So, you learned lessons about life that you never thought you'd have to learn," I said.

"Yes, you wouldn't choose to learn them in the manner that we did, but we have worked hard to be positive, and to move forward," Kim said.

Olivia grew tired of the chips and the conversation. She distracted Kevin for a moment as she decided which movie she wanted to watch for the hundredth time. Once more, she looked directly at me as her words came blasting through. She held the movie up for my inspection, and when I agreed with her choice, she moved to the living room and sat down in her Barbie chair.

"She's beautiful," I said.

"One other change in our life is that we pray together each night before going to sleep. We thank God for each other, and we say an Our Father and think of Chaplain Betty and the influence she had in our lives," Kim said.

"Where do you stand in regard to Olivia's health? You had mentioned that it was possible that she would face another surgery down the line."

"Well, Olivia just went for a speech evaluation, and it looks like she will need speech therapy," Kim said. "There is a chance that a second surgery, called a pharyngeal flap surgery, may be required. We will start with the therapy and go from there."

"We'll be a total wreck before another surgical procedure,"

Kevin added. "But we'll face it together. We know for sure that Olivia will put up a good fight, no matter what she faces."

"She's a tough little girl," I said.

"That's what's amazing," Kim said. "Olivia's strength and will to fight are the main reasons why she got through that horrible situation. She is extremely strong-willed and determined. Before she was in the coma, she fought every step of the way by ripping away the oxygen mask. Even when she was in the coma, she fought. Her blood pressure would rise in anger each time they tried to shift her into a new position. On the day she came off the ventilator, Omar explained to us that he didn't have a choice. He even called her a beast that night."

"I know, as we wrap this up, that you have a number of people that you'd like to thank."

"We are eternally grateful to our families, "Kevin said," but we also feel as if our family was extended by our stay at The Women and Children's Hospital."

"Dr. Omar and Kathy LaJudice played a huge role in our time at PICU. They completely supported us as well as Olivia. They became our friends," Kim said.

"And you speak about Family-Centered Care, Dr. Budi and Dr. Omar could be the poster-doctors for that initiative," Kevin added. "They treated us as a family. They weren't simply treating medical symptoms. We were truly involved in the care of our child. The doctors would show us the X-ray's and explain the situation. We can't say enough about the way that they treated our daughter and us. They were just wonderful."

"We also had a truly special bond with Kathy LaJudice. She was Olivia's nurse on nearly every day that she worked and she not only took care of Olivia, she took care of us. Lynn was the recovery room nurse who came to visit Olivia every day for a week after the surgery. Dr. Chudy stopped by each and every day. It simply blew our minds that these people took time out of their days to come and visit with Olivia even when she was out of their direct care."

"Those are the things you learn," Kevin said. "What would

have been easy for us was to just place blame and feel anger and rage. What we found instead was a lot of love and thoughtfulness that we will carry with us every day for the rest of our lives."

Kim and Kevin didn't have to say much more. Their gratitude was overwhelming. Their grace in the face of pressure was admirable, and the love that they have developed, as a family, was heartwarming.

Almost on cue, Olivia returned from the living room. She jumped into Kevin's arms and he placed a quick kiss on the side of her angelic face. "We were lucky," Kevin whispered.

Kim took in the entire scene. She did her best to fight off the emotion of the moment, but a couple of stray tears developed in the corners of her eyes. "Our daughter is a special little girl. God saved her because she has a lot more to do in this life. Olivia will do anything that she puts her mind to. We were very lucky."

As I gathered up my notebooks and stood up, Olivia made sure that I will always remember how beautiful her story is. She summed it all up for me by flashing her terrific smile.

CHAPTER 19

The Story of Dr. Michael Caty
Part II

*"If what you're working for really matters,
you'll give it all you got."*
—Nido Qubein

One of the final tasks on my to-do list in regard to care at The Women and Children's Hospital was to take a guided tour of the facility with Dr. Michael Caty. My inspiration behind such a tour was simple; I needed the professional hand of a man who knew every corner of the hospital and could explain what was being done on a daily basis. Our walk-through took place on a cold November day just before Thanksgiving. I entered Dr. Caty's office with the excitement of learning even more about how business was conducted on a daily basis, but was most surprised to find out that what I had learned during the writing of this book would be simply reinforced in our walk-through.

The first stop on our tour was the front door of the pediatric surgery/operating room. The brightly-painted walls and the well-lit hallway belied my image of an operating room as a dark, scary place where children's lives hang in the balance.

"There are two specialized operating rooms that are available for the performance of miniature access surgery," Dr. Caty explained. "We've had the miniature access surgery center for about five years now, and approximately 80% of all surgeries are performed using laporoscopy. All of the pediatric surgeons in North America were trained here, and the equipment available to us is state-of-the-art. Children are not just small adults. The equipment and the surgical techniques used here are designed to meet the special needs of every child. The Women & Children's Hospital is the only hospital in the region to have pediatric surgical sub-specialists for dental medicine, neurosurgery, ophthalmology, orthopedics, otolaryngology, urology, and general pediatric surgery. An operating room with specialized radiography equipment is used for patients followed by the Breast Care Center."

"Having the proper equipment has made your life easier, I imagine," I said.

"We're one of the top five or six best-equipped surgical units in the country," Dr. Caty said. "Let's head to Variety-8."

As we walked through the halls, Dr. Caty addressed each person that passed with a smile and a first-name greeting. It entered my mind that learning medical terms would be difficult enough, but I was walking with a man who not only educated himself through the years, but also remembered the name of each person walking the halls of the hospital.

"Variety-8 is home to a completely renovated 22-bed Hematology/Oncology Unit. It is an inpatient unit for children diagnosed with cancer, blood disorders, and other medical conditions. The unit was designed to better accommodate patients and their families who have extended and frequent follow-up stays."

We stepped off the elevator and walked down the hall to the nurse's station. "Good morning," Dr. Caty said to the nurse.

The Child Life playroom directly across from the nurse's station diverted my attention. A boy of about four years of age was working a train around a track. The boy was dressed in a light green hospital gown. His right arm was heavily bandaged, but my eyes went to the over-sized beige socks on his feet. He barely glanced up as we entered the room.

"The Child Life playroom is like a sanctuary for the children," Dr. Caty said. "I try my best not to enter the room on a regular basis because it is like a safe zone for the children. It's a place where they can play, free of worries about their medical care."

Deena, a Child Life Specialist, smiled at me. "Hey, buddy," she said to the boy. "Do you want me to fix your socks?"

The boy smiled at Deena, and then turned to look at me. His big brown eyes met mine, and he smiled quickly before turning his attention back to his train.

"Good morning, Bessie," Dr. Caty said. He moved to the center of the room and smiled at a slender, middle-aged woman who was wiping down some of the other toys in the room. "Bessie is a volunteer who provides an invaluable service around here."

Bessie smiled broadly as Dr. Caty addressed her.

"How long have you been coming to the hospital as a volunteer?" Dr. Caty asked.

"Seventeen years," Bessie answered. "I am a volunteer through the foster grandparent program. I come by five days a week."

"How far away do you live?" Dr. Caty asked.

"About fifteen miles," Bessie answered.

"Thank you for the work you do," I said.

"I enjoy it tremendously," Bessie said.

It was difficult to imagine such a commitment. Bessie was a true superstar in my eyes. I had started the tour believing I would be a witness to the magic of healthcare, and the simple magic of it all was displayed in the giving spirit of people like Bessie and Deena.

"The unit is a comfortable environment for the families of long-term patients. Some of the suites are equipped with private showers. The parent lounge has a kitchenette, a television, and couch and chairs that offer a comfortable environment for a family to rest in privacy without leaving the floor on which their child is admitted. Patients and their families can be very loyal to a specific floor."

Dr. Caty led the way down the hallway toward the elevators once more. "The 9th floor is for sameday surgery care."

We stepped off the elevator and my eyes were immediately drawn to the beautiful dolphin paintings displayed on the floor. Dr. Caty led the way by the bulletin board with photos of the Care team. Dr. Caty followed my eyes to the impressive display.

"One of the things that we decided to do was to display the photos of the Care team so that families could put a name to a face. It's a subtle thing, but when you're a patient here, it is easier if you know whom you are dealing with."

Photos of the pastoral staff, the residents and the general surgery team were prominently displayed. We walked further down the hall, and I took note of the Kaleida Health Family bulletin board that displayed tips for patients and staff members alike.

"This is a new display too," I said.

"It is all a part of the initiative that we have been heading toward for the last three years," Dr. Caty said. "If a family is better informed about what is happening, then it becomes a little easier to provide positive care. For the past three years we've been working on collaborative surgical rounds. It's a practice that is common at adult hospitals, but we are one of the only children's hospitals that have initiated the practice. The collaborative surgical rounds are a commitment that we made to establish a practice of being well-informed about a patient. The rounds include the attending residents, the office staff, the physical therapist, the nurses and the pharmacists. We will discuss the particulars of a patient's care with the family present. We will present vital signs and, to include them in the process, will ask the family, 'Is that right?' We will read the list of prescribed medicines and discuss the plans that are being made. It is a practice that allows everyone to be informed about the patient, but it also provides a measure of safety, as the pharmacist is also present and can verify the medicines necessary. The main purpose of the collaborative rounds program, however, is to provide excellence in care."

"The cost of doing the collaborative rounds and all of the improvements must be tremendous," I said. "As I've worked on this story, it has become apparent to me that the care that families expect and deserve has to be paid for."

"There's no question that rising healthcare costs are an issue," Dr. Caty said. "But what we are doing is vitally important to each and every family. Our goal is to provide optimum care. For instance, in your son's case, we tried to anticipate and prepare. Before Jake's operation, we had a plan for care, but we also prepared a Plan B, Plan C, and Plan D. Say, for example, that we had begun the surgery *without* preparing for ECMO care if it had been needed. The results may be very different if we do not prepare for what might be necessary. To put it in explainable terms, it is important to bring a gun to a knife fight if necessary."

Our conversation was briefly interrupted by the appearance of a boy of about ten or eleven years old. The boy, who was in a wheelchair, with a cast on his right leg, appeared in the door of his room, and immediately caught Dr. Caty's attention. "Good morning, Cody," Dr. Caty said. "Are you ready to go home?"

"Yes!" Cody answered enthusiastically.

"That's great," Dr. Caty replied. "You did a super job."

Cody smiled. Very subtly, Dr. Caty touched the boy's right arm. "You take care of yourself, okay?"

"I will," Cody answered.

We drifted back toward the elevators. "Let's visit the NICU."

"You know what?" I asked. "The entire hospital seems more inviting to me. When I was here, it seemed darker somehow. Every floor seems brighter and more comfortable somehow. Perhaps it's because I don't have a child in an emergency situation, but am I wrong?"

"No, we've made a number of improvements in the last five years. We are all about making families feel more comfortable now. We certainly want to work to that end."

We exited the elevator and headed toward the beautiful, recently redone NICU. I had toured the unit while interviewing Linda Eschberger and Sue Popenberg. Just before we entered the unit a question that I had asked Dr. Feldman leapt to mind. "When we spoke the first time, I neglected to ask you, when you're performing an operation, are you actually afraid? I mean that's an awfully crude way to put it, but as a human being, are you fearful of what can happen?"

"Of course," Dr. Caty said. "When you're doing an operation, there are major concerns that must be addressed. As the operation moves forward, there are additional concerns that present themselves. It's a matter of breaking down the operation to tasks that can be handled. There are always new concerns to address, but as you move on in your career, the list of surgeries that you haven't seen before is shortened."

We toured the NICU, following much the same path that I had followed when speaking with Linda and Sue.

"The NICU is one of the largest in the United States," Dr. Caty said. "It is a unit that we can certainly be proud of."

"I'm amazed with the work that goes on here," I said.

"It's a completely unique discipline," Dr. Caty observed. "The unit is responsible for long-term care. In a lot of ways, the nurses are like foster parents for some of the children who must be here for a long time."

The final step on our tour was the PICU. As we stepped off the elevator at the 2nd floor, we met up with Dr. Stanley Lau and Dr. Celeste Hollands. Of course, Dr. Caty's greeting was enthusiastic. He introduced me and told the doctors of my intention to write the story of the hospital.

"Seriously?" Dr. Lau asked. "That's great! What would make you write a story about the hospital?"

"My intentions are to shine some light on the team of people who work here," I said.

"That is terrific," Dr. Hollands said. "We aren't looking for attention for the job we do, but it's nice that you've noticed."

Moments later, Dr. Caty and I stood in the center of the PICU. It was a place that I was all too familiar with from Jake's time at the hospital. It was also a place where I almost felt comfortable, in a strange sort of way. The care that Jake and hundreds of others before him had received in the PICU was nothing short of amazing.

"The unit is busy for twenty-four hours out of every day," Dr. Caty said. "The PICU operates with speed, efficiency, and expertise around the clock."

We stopped in the center of the unit. Doctors and nurses moved from room to room, and I simply allowed my eyes to follow their hurried movements. My glance stopped at room number four, where Jake had spent his most trying of days. I didn't say anything, but my heart filled with gratitude at the thought that the people I had interviewed, and hundreds of others on staff at the hospital, were willing to lead quiet lives of dignity and service.

Dr. Caty led me out of the unit and down the hall toward his office. I was mindful of not wanting to take up much more of his time, but he had been more than accommodating. "By virtue of being here, each and every child is a personality," he began. "The true celebrities in your story are the children. Say for instance that Abigail visits the hospital for care. The clerk at the desk on the floor where she is admitted will know her name. As a surgeon, I will be able to walk up to that clerk and say, 'How's Abigail?' and that clerk will know whom I am talking about. The Child Life Department will meet Abigail and know her name and personality. Brian Smistek will take Abigail's photo, and will get to know Abigail and why she is here. During Leadership Rounds, Cheryl Klass will meet Abigail. Each of the nurses who work with Abigail will understand how she likes to be treated. The security guards at the front desk will recognize Abigail's family. Colleen Hurley, the nurse practitioner, will meet Abigail, and will work with her to ensure that the level of care is optimal. The respiratory therapist and the anesthesiologist may meet with Abigail and her family. Cheryl, the cashier in the cafeteria, will recognize Abigail's family. In all, from the time she comes in to the end of her stay, Abigail may meet 200 to 300 people who know her name and are working toward taking care of her problem. That is the type of healthcare that we are striving for. The celebrities of your story are the children like Abigail. We are all just a part of a team that cares for her."

As I shook Dr. Caty's hand and thanked him for his time, his beeper went off. He glanced down at the unit and headed toward his phone. "It's always good to see you," he said.

I headed out the side door and exited onto Hodge Street. As I walked toward the parking ramp, I passed by at least half a dozen children who were about to get the full celebrity treatment. I turned around and looked up at the building. Before my child got sick, The Women & Children's Hospital was simply a building. Now, I knew that it was so much more. *Thank God that Buffalo has such a place*, I thought. *Thank God for the people who work inside.*

CHAPTER 20

The Story of Alexia Grace Kilroy

"Live for today, but hold your hands open to tomorrow.
Anticipate the future and its changes with joy.
There is a seed of God's love in every event, every unpleasant
situation in which you may find yourself."
—*Barbara Johnson*

What would you be willing to do for love? Through the years, men and women have proclaimed their love for their children by saying that they would walk across hot burning coals for them, or scale the highest mountain. Millions of mothers explain that they would do anything and everything to keep their children safe from harm. Alexia Grace Kilroy was born into this world, because of the tremendous devotion and dedication of a very special family and a mother who was willing to climb the highest mountain and swim the deepest sea. For Alexia, born on February 7, 2006, a story of love was being written as she developed into the beautiful girl who she is today.

I met with Brooke Kilroy on a bitterly cold winter day. Her daughter, Alexia, was mere weeks away from celebrating her first birthday. Brooke introduced me to her daughter, who eyed me suspiciously. "She's a little leery of strangers," Brooke said, "but she'll come around."

Brooke led me into the beautiful, spacious home she shared with her husband Mark and Alexia. She handed Alexia off to her grandmother, Betty Diemert, who was thrilled with the idea of spending time with the child. I smiled at Alexia once more, and our eyes locked for a brief moment before she turned away. It didn't take anymore than a second to see the astounding beauty of this sweet girl.

"I'm going to try and get through this without crying too much," Brooke said, and in that statement, I felt the amazing bond of love between a mother and a child. "I'm the oldest of six children. As I grew up, my family was always at the center of my life. When Mark and I were married, starting our own family was very important."

Yet starting a family proved to be anything but routine. As a young woman, Brooke Kilroy was diagnosed with cervical cancer. Thankfully, Brooke was able to fend off the second most common cancer among women. While complications are generally uncommon, the young couple understood that women who are able to conceive after surgery are prone to pre-term labor or possible late-term miscarriage.

"We understood there were risks associated with the pregnancy," Brooke said. "Yet we were extremely careful. Every two weeks, Dr. Laurel White examined me. We went through many sonograms that did not show any changes, so we thought we were going to be lucky and not have any problems."

Brooke's eyes threatened tears as she described the crucial moment of the pregnancy. "Then I had a routine doctor's appointment scheduled for October 26th. I'm not sure why, but the night before the appointment, I woke up crying. There wasn't any reason for my tears, but I just knew that something was wrong. I felt great, but without any reason whatsoever, I was scared to go to that appointment."

Brooke's terror was well founded. "As the technician performed the sonogram, I kept my fears bottled up inside, but almost immediately, I understood there was a problem. The technician looked at the screen and said, 'Oh, that doesn't look good.'"

The technician alerted Dr. White, who very calmly explained to Brooke that her cervix was funneling. "The weight of the baby was pushing the cervix open from the inside out. Dr. White explained it to me, and while I was scared, her low-key demeanor calmed me. I was scheduled to return to work. At the time, I was working as a psychologist at Niagara University. Dr. White explained that it would be okay if I returned to work to clear my schedule for the next day, but for some reason, I decided against going in. Dr. White explained she would confer with my obstetrician, Dr. Roger Schneider, and she would likely see me in her office next week after some bed rest. Yet, rather than heading to the university, I went home and got hold of my family. While I was home, I received a call from Dr. Schneider's office. I was told to lie down right away, and it was explained to me that he had arranged an appointment at The Women & Children's Hospital of Buffalo. Mark and I rushed to the hospital, and I was admitted to the labor and delivery unit. I was still believing that I was visiting the hospital simply to be checked out, or for a second opinion, but in reality, they were concerned I would deliver the baby that night." Brooke sighed heavily and we both took a sip of water. "That's not to say I was cognizant of the true emergency of the situation." Her eyes welled with tears and she professed the sentiment that I've grown accustomed to hearing. "I grew up in the area and I remember hearing about the hospital and the wonderful people who work there, but there truly is no sense of appreciation until you need help. I don't think I could have made it without the support of the hospital staff."

"How far into the pregnancy were you?" I asked.

"I had carried the baby for twenty-five weeks and six days," Brooke said. "The neo-natal doctor explained that the baby wasn't viable if carried less than twenty-six weeks. I understood that *viable* meant that, if I were to deliver on that day, my baby wouldn't live."

Brooke's voice faded a bit as she said the words. Instinctively she looked to the room where Alexia was playing with Brooke's grandmother. A slight smile creased Brooke's lips and she allowed me a glimpse into the love that she feels. "They put me on a monitor to feel for the contractions and the baby's heartbeat.

I was heading straight into labor, and the staff worked hard to administer meds to stave off the labor. They provided steroids that would work to develop the baby's lungs. At that point I was in total shock. I was afraid that the baby was going to die, and some of the staff seemed to be preparing me for that outcome. It was explained that if I were to deliver, there was a high probability of severe problems. If I were to carry the baby for another week, the probability would decrease. That's the mindset I worked hard to develop. I needed to hold the baby. I would have to do whatever was necessary to make sure that the baby would develop."

A look of fierce determination crossed Brooke's face. Just as I was allowed a look at her love for Alexia, I was also being granted a glimpse of a mother's tremendous resolve.

"My family responded, of course. My mother, Marlene, and father, Robert, were right beside me. Of course, Mark was there, feeling all of it with me, but what really got to me were my siblings. One of my sisters, Ashley, left school at Penn State and arrived at the hospital at four in the morning. Ashley petitioned some of her friends to go to her classes to take notes so that she could be with me. My sister Christen flew in from Tennessee. It was a family moment, to be sure, and everyone was there for us."

"Through it all, the staff was telling you what to expect?" I asked.

"Oh, it was all laid out for me. I understood that the goal was to make it through the milestones set before me. It was literally one day at a time. I knew the twenty-six week guidepost was important, and once I achieved that, we talked about making it to the twenty-seventh week. I was on strict bed rest, which meant that I had to lie totally flat. I couldn't even raise the bed an inch. I was allowed to stand only to go to the bathroom. I was allowed to sit at the sink for five minutes each day. I could raise the bed for a half-hour after meals so that I could digest properly, but I wasn't comfortable doing that and I normally laid flat well before the half hour was up."

"That's incredible," I whispered. "What were you thinking?"

"I couldn't focus on anything very well," Brooke said. "I found that I didn't have the concentration to read an entire magazine article or watch half an hour of television. I just kept telling myself I needed to be there and that I would do what I needed to do. It sounds funny, but my goal was simply to stay in the hospital, flat on my back, so my baby could develop."

"Did you talk to her?" I asked.

"I did speak to the baby," Brooke said, "but we didn't know it was a her yet. Through all of the sonograms and all of the tests, we didn't know that we were having a daughter. Mark and I wanted it to be a surprise, and we held to that."

"And through it all, you worked with the staff to ensure that things remained stable."

"I was having contractions every day," Brooke said. "They weren't painful, but they were constant. There was plenty of activity around me. The residents were in and out all day, every day, and I quickly became friends with the nursing staff. There were three doctors on rotation, Dr. Amol Lele, Dr. Bruce Rodgers, and Dr. Jack Lawler. Each doctor was fully aware of where we were and how the baby was developing inside of me. I settled into a routine of sorts, but I'm not sure if I would've made it through without the love of my family and the love of the staff. Everyone was so incredible."

"And still, you endured, one day at a time."

"One moment at a time," Brooke said with a laugh. "There were frustrations, of course. I couldn't shower or wash. A certified medical assistant, Angelique "Angie" Lee, would wash my hair once or a twice a week, and that was such a wonderful moment. My gosh, I looked forward to that so much."

Brooke inched forward in her chair and as her gaze wandered her eyes glistened with tears once more. "The sweet things that people did for me fill my heart with gratitude. The Director of Women's Services, Julie Polka, was always asking me if there was anything that she could do to make me more comfortable. They put a magazine rack right next to my bed so that I could just grab a magazine when I needed to. It might seem like a small thing, but not when you're just lying there. Marcia Sarkin, Director of Volunteers for Women's Services, stopped by weekly with cookies or knitting needles or anything they could think of. It made me realize that they weren't just doing their jobs, but that they truly cared about my baby and me. I made life-long friends, and it's so hard to express how thankful we are."

"Slowly, the days turned to weeks," I said.

"Very slowly," Brooke answered with a laugh. "I was on pins and needles all the time, and every once in awhile I was in sheer panic, believing that the baby would be coming. There were at least two or three instances when the Labor and Delivery staff were called to my room because they were sure that I wouldn't be able to stave off the birth any longer."

"Yet you did. Day after day, week after week, you carried that child. Flat on your back with no more respite than about a half an hour a day, you did what you needed to do."

"We all did what we needed to do," Brooke corrected me. "Mark was incredible. It was so hard on him too. He was driving from work to the hospital and back home. He was supportive and soothing and completely stressed out, but he didn't show that to me. He was there every day, but he set Friday night up as date night. He would bring dinner and stay over with me."

Again, Brooke's eyes were home to tears. She shrugged and smiled the tears away. "I find that I become overwhelmed when I think about what everyone did for me. My mom, for instance, was amazing. She was there each and everyday, and she would stay most of the day. She decorated my room and my bathroom. She hung posters and put flowers and a rug in the bathroom. People from the hospital would bring other patients by to tour my room. It was incredible. My father would work all day and then come to visit, bringing my favorite oatmeal cookies from the café. My aunt, Dianne Beirne, was there to give me backrubs. My co-workers not only handled my workload, but they stopped by to keep me company."

One such co-worker, Kathy Palazzo, would cry each and every time that she spoke to her friend. Brooke's brothers and brother-in-law would visit faithfully. Her mother and father-in-law sent a card every day. Prayers were being said all across the Western New York area. Chaplain Betty DiVito would bring communion to Brooke and pray with her on a regular basis. "When you're in a situation that you don't have a lot of control over, you rely on faith," Brooke said.

Remarkably, Brooke was able to sustain the pregnancy. At thirty-five weeks, Brooke was sent home from The Women & Children's Hospital of Buffalo.

Just as we are about to discuss her birth, Alexia crawled into the room. She was dressed in a beautiful pink nightgown. She was still eyeing me suspiciously, but when she turned to her mother, she smiled. Betty gathered up Alexia and returned her to the room just off the kitchen. Alexia could still see me, however, and she stared at me just as my children had done when they were babies. Perhaps she could sense my true wonder and awe. Before too long, she tired of my adoring glance.

"You must have been relieved to be getting out of that hospital bed," I said.

"Actually, what was truly incredible was I was afraid to be go home for the rest of my pregnancy. I had become so close to the staff that I was a little frightened to be leaving them. I had spent the holidays in the hospital. On Thanksgiving and Christmas, my family had come to the hospital with food and gifts. The nursing staff had packed my room and made me feel at home. It was a holiday season that I'll never forget. It was almost as though we had a larger family to share the season with."

"Describe what it felt like to be leaving the hospital at thirty-five weeks."

"The day before I left the hospital, I was allowed to walk around a little bit. After being flat on my back for so long, it was actually a strange sensation. I didn't want to do too much though, and on the way home, I lay in the back of the car. When I arrived home, the transition was a little difficult. I was sort of on my own for medications. I had to learn to give myself a shot."

Brooke's eyes threatened tears once more and I could almost

sense that it was gratitude that was once again causing the swell of emotion. "The most difficult aspect of it all was that I found myself missing everyone at the hospital. My mom was at the house every day, and it was wonderful to be around Mark and the home again, but I found myself thinking about my new friends at the hospital. I was still scared, and a little disappointed that I couldn't do some of the things that a typical first-time mother could do. Mark worked hard to set things up for the arrival of the baby, but I wanted to go to Babies 'R Us, you know?"

"Yet being in your own home had to be more comfortable."

"Yes and no," Brooke said. "Of course we were thrilled that the baby had made it through the most difficult of times, but there was still a tremendous amount of fear. I was still seeing Dr. Amol Lele on a weekly basis. I remained on my back for most of the next three weeks, but I began to imagine how we would get to the hospital and what might happen if we didn't have enough time."

Brooke's water broke at three o'clock on the morning of February 7, 2006. On the way to the hospital, Brooke contacted Nurse Mary Jo Murphy from the high-risk pregnancy unit. "Mary Jo was always there for me," Brooke said. "When I was flat on my back, Mary Jo would visit me when she wasn't even scheduled to be at work. On the day of delivery, she came in to be with me in the labor and delivery unit. Years before, my grandfather, who was a veterinarian in Lockport, Dr. Ralph Lewis, had saved a kitten for the Murphy family. My grandfather hadn't charged for the work, and Mary Jo thought that was the greatest thing in the world. She found it ironic that years and years later, she was helping me through the birth of my 'kitten'. Yet, just like grandpa, she was doing more than what was expected. She was doing so much more than just her job."

Brooke's voice trailed off. In the other room, Alexia laughed at something that her great grandmother had said. We both turned in the direction of the room. "Oh yeah, the birth," Brooke said. "After speaking with Mary Jo, I paged ahead to Judette Dahleiden, the Manager of the Mother and Baby Unit and High-

Risk Pregnancy floor. Judette called ahead to the hospital. It was interesting because the drive in was anything but typical. Mark had to negotiate his way through a nasty snowstorm, but when we finally got to the hospital the nurse greeted us by saying, 'That's great! We heard you were coming in.' It was just unbelievable that the entire staff was excited too."

"Were there any complications?"

"Actually, it was a fairly routine birth. There was a moment when we became concerned because the cord was wrapped around the baby's neck, but it all went well."

Brooke's eyes flashed a hint of relief, coupled with the excitement of a day that she will vividly recall forever. "During the birth process, it was difficult to feel excitement. It was strange to be pushing the baby to come out after I had spent so much time trying to keep her in."

"I recall the exact moment of my children's births," I said. "That had to be a magical moment."

"Unbelievable! It really is a miracle," Brooke said. "It was two minutes after four in the afternoon, and the level of excitement in the ward was something you could almost feel. The staff had worked up a pool for the exact moment of the birth. Channel 7 News reported on the delivery, and the hospital photographer, Brian Smistek, was there to take a number of wonderful photographs. Some of the nurses brought gifts for the baby."

"And now, you have the beautiful family that you had always dreamed about."

Brooke smiled and turned to look at Alexia, who was in a small swing, oblivious to the fear, and ultimate happiness, that she brought to her young family. "Looking back, it doesn't seem like it was so hard to do. It was what my baby needed me to do. I'd do anything for her now, too. It's a great thing to be blessed with such a capacity for love. The nursing staff and I used to joke that I had a faulty door to the oven, or that we just needed the baby to incubate a little longer."

Brooke offered a truly sweet laugh that I am happy to share.

"Are you thinking about having another child?" I asked.

Brooke rolled her eyes, but incredibly she explained that the subject has been thoroughly discussed with Mark and a trusted medical staff.

"Maybe there won't be any problems," I said.

"Oh, there'll be problems," Brooke replied. "But, gosh, it's worth it."

As I grabbed my notebook and headed toward the door, Brooke gathered Alexia, and together they saw me off. As I was putting on my boots to head back into the wild winter afternoon, Alexia offered her one and only smile to me. "I knew she'd loosen up," Brooke said.

I drove down the long, winding driveway away from the Kilroy home. Alexia's beautiful smile and Brooke's final words were fighting for space inside my head. Alexia's smile would be easy enough to remember, as she was a beautiful girl, born into a world of love. Yet it was Brooke's final words that echoed for a long time as I drove down the road toward home. "Make sure that you write that we couldn't have made it without the love of our families and the love of the wonderful staff at The Women & Children's Hospital of Buffalo."

CHAPTER 21

The Story of Cheryl Klass, President of Women & Children's Hospital of Buffalo

"We are what we repeatedly do.
Excellence, then, is not an act but a habit."
— *Aristotle*

As I stood near the administration offices awaiting my appointment with Women & Children's Hospital of Buffalo President Cheryl Klass, my eyes drifted to the bulletin board to the left of the door. At the very top of the board were the words: "The Voice of WCHOB—what do our patients, families and co-workers have to say?"

There were words of encouragement and recognition for the men and women working at the hospital, but what caught my eye, more than anything else, was a hand-written note from an obviously young child. The handwriting was jumbled and there were cross-outs on the sheet. As I began to read, I felt the complete grace and innocence of the child author.

> *Dear Children's Hospital,*
> *My name is Elena. A few of my friends and I went around our neighborhood and collected money for some of the children in your hospital. We felt sad that so many children are sick in the*

*hospital so we wanted to make them feel better and my other
friends are named Rachel and Kiana. I hope this helps.*
    Sincerely,
    Elena, Kiana and Rachel

With my heart firmly planted in my throat, I entered the administration office for my meeting with Cheryl Klass. By all accounts, Cheryl Klass is a remarkable woman with a true vision for what the hospital can be.

Rosanne Radigan, the administrative secretary, escorted me into Cheryl's office. The interview had been at least three months in the making, having been postponed by the Buffalo weather and our busy schedules. Rosanne apologized for the delay in setting up the meeting, but I explained that it had actually worked to my advantage. Interviewing Cheryl at the outset would have been completely different from interviewing her after I had the chance to speak with her staff.

Cheryl met us at the door to her office. She offered a warm, inviting smile that I had recognized from each and every face-to-face meeting. Cheryl had been extremely supportive of the release of *Counting on a Miracle*, and as much as I admired her work, she offered me the same sort of respect.

"Thank you for taking the time to meet with me," Cheryl said. She offered me a seat at a small conference table in the corner of her office. I scanned the neatly decorated, well-kept office. "Thank you," I said. "Before we get started on your story, I feel like I have to tell you how positive the feeling is around the hospital. You have a staff of people who respect and admire your work, and as the father of a former patient, I have to tell you that things have certainly changed in the five years since my son was treated here."

"Thank you, I do hope the morale is better. How is Jake?"

I thought of Dr. Caty's words stating that a child was a celebrity to the staff, just by virtue of being a patient at the hospital. "Jake is wonderful," I said. "He's very healthy, and he's probably driving his mother nuts right now."

"Great, that's what he's supposed to be doing," Cheryl said.

Like each and every member of the staff, Cheryl seemed a bit uncomfortable with my attention to the hospital. While she was thrilled with my acknowledgement that there was a truly positive vibe working in the halls of the hospital, Cheryl was not in the business of accepting praise for the work that she believed was essential. The attitude in the hospital had changed during Cheryl's tenure simply because it was the best way to do business.

"So, this is your story," I said. "Each and every person I interviewed cites your communication skills and unbelievable passion for the job. How did you get here?"

Cheryl offered a comfortable smile. It was a smile that thanked me for my kind words and summed up her long journey to the chair of president.

"When I was in the 9th grade, I came to the hospital to visit a friend who had major spinal surgery. While I was here, I was impressed with the care and dedication of the staff that was helping my friend. The nurses were simply wonderful. They were calm, tender, and caring. They made eye contact as they administered care. I knew right then and there that I wanted to be a nurse who helped others. I finished high school and studied nursing at Niagara University. In 1977, I returned to the hospital as a nurse, and I was in awe of the incredible staff of people who were here. To be honest, I just wanted to work here. I just wanted to make the cut." Cheryl laughed nervously.

"Almost everyone whom I've spoken with knew this was where they wanted to spend their career. Is that how it was for you?" I asked.

"Certainly, but there were a few twists along the way. I was very happy being a part of the nursing staff here, and saw myself in that capacity for years, but when I had the opportunity to become the nurse manager, I accepted because I felt I was in a better position to have an impact in patient care. From there, I became the director of pediatrics and pediatric care and ultimately the chief nursing officer, but in 1995, I relocated with my husband and children to Chicago. It was very difficult to leave, but it was the right move for our family."

During her time at Children's Memorial Hospital in Chicago, Cheryl continued to pursue her career goals with little thought that she would someday sit in the chair of the president of the hospital that she loved. Cheryl obtained an MBA from the Kellogg School at Northwestern University. Her tenure at Children's Memorial Hospital included appointments as the chief nursing officer and the chief operating officer. All the while, Cheryl worked with her husband, Geoff, to raise three daughters, Erin, Catherine, and Ann.

"That's a remarkable body of work," I said softly.

"It seems that way now," Cheryl said, "but at the time there wasn't any sort of grand plan. We were working hard, but I truly wasn't thinking that I would be the president of The Women & Children's Hospital of Buffalo. I was a working nurse with an idea of what made for the type of care that was provided for my friend back when I was in the 9th grade."

Cheryl's twisting, turning career lead to a return to Buffalo where she worked as chief operating officer at Sister's Hospital and Mercy Hospital. In June of 2004, Cheryl was appointed as President of Women and Children's.

"That is a wild ride," I said. "Yet you must have been unbelievably thrilled."

"Certainly. I was excited with the opportunity because I knew that the core team was still very much intact. The hospital had endured some challenging times. In 2002 there was the actual threat of closure, and there were changes implemented by the Kaleida Health team. The staff was a little uncertain about the direction of the hospital, but I felt that the core group of people assembled here would be able to recognize the strengths. I felt that we were in a good position to celebrate what happens here on a daily basis."

"Personally speaking, how do you handle the challenge of the endless parade of sick children?" I asked.

"It's what we do," Cheryl said. "The human side of it is that we see parents in their most fearful, vulnerable position. Personally, I've always gained strength from watching the amazing bond between a parent and a child, and the equally important bond between the child and the caregiver."

"Was it more difficult to see sick children when you became a mother?"

"Oh yeah," Cheryl said. "I remember one operation where I didn't want to take a child from his mother."

"There are certain aspects of leadership and management that must be exercised in order to boost morale and make effective changes," I said. "As I noted, there appears to be a more comfortable working environment at the hospital now. Given the fact that your tenure began after the proposed closure of the hospital and some very difficult times, it must have been difficult to implement the necessary changes."

"As far as leadership goes, you're only as good as the people around you, at every level. I'm fortunate to be working at a hospital where the doctors and nurses share my passion for work in pediatrics. I appreciate that the morale seems heightened, and it is certainly how we would like to work, but when I returned here, we worked hard to focus on a more narrow group of projects. We identified areas where we wanted to improve, and we specifically targeted four main areas. The areas we targeted included Cardiac Surgery, and the hard work of Dr. Michael Caty and Dr. Dan Pieroni was instrumental in the achievement of our goals. Another targeted area was Neurosciences, and the staff responsible for advancement included Dr. Frank Schreck, Dr. Veetai Li, Dr. Frederick Munschauer III, and Dr. Curtis Rozzelle. The third area that we targeted was OB/Neonatal Care, and changes were highlighted by the work of Dr. Ivan D'Souza, and Dr. Rita Ryan. In Hematology/Oncology, Dr. Martin Brecher led the charge."

"Let me get this right," I said. "You worked to make changes in these focused areas, believing that it would change the entire feel of care at the hospital?"

Cheryl nodded. "The doctors involved were extremely focused and determined. Also, there were tremendous capital investments made in the building, and we regained some of the lost volume and market share through future planning and by regaining the confidence of the community."

"The tremendous growth and change seemed to come from within. Is there a single thing that you can attribute that to?"

"Passion," Cheryl said without hesitation. "There are so many people who are extremely passionate about the work they do here. I mentioned each of those doctors in the targeted areas, but there are so many more people who make it all work on a daily basis. You can't manufacture the passion of people like Mary Ellen Creighton, or Kathy Humphrey, or Elsie Dawe, or Joanne Lana, or Barb Kourkounis. I can actually name about a hundred people off the top of my head."

"So could I," I said, and we laughed.

"My job is to match the people with passion to the right area, and to make sure that the resources are available."

"You mentioned the Buffalo community," I said.

"It's wonderful," Cheryl said. "The foundations, the corporate sponsorships, the dedicated donors and the wonderful volunteers. It's simply an exceptional community."

"Yet, when you speak about leadership, you seem to be doing what each and every person here does. You're deflecting my praise and passing it on to the staff of people that work around you. Your changes must be reflected in the work you do."

"We are certainly a team, and as administrators, we are simply one aspect of the entire operation. As a member of the team, we need to be accessible to the nursing staff, the doctors, and the patients. On a daily basis we conduct Leadership Rounds where we visit a specific department, meet with staff, and the patients. Recognizing that the hospital isn't just operational from nine to five on weekdays, we also conduct leadership rounds on evenings and weekends. When I first started back here, I would come through the hospital on a Saturday, and I would get some looks as people wondered why I was there. Now, I don't get those looks so often, so I've been here on a lot of Saturdays."

"What is the end result of the Leadership Rounds?" I asked.

"The rounds present a true sense of purpose. We're able to

identify problems that a specific department might be having. We've initiated communication forums within the department so that we can answer the 'what if' questions, and so that we can implement thoughtful solutions."

"Leadership is then consistent and effectively communicated," I said.

"Exactly," Cheryl said, "and we are open and accessible to staff members. It also gives me the chance to see the patients, the parents, and the wonderful families. You asked about the endless parade of sick children that is part of the job, but I am remotivated on a daily basis from seeing the families…and the newborns!"

With the mere mention of the newborns, Cheryl was out of her chair. She moved to her desk and quickly retrieved a tiny t-shirt. The small garment was baby blue and bore the words, "I was born at Women & Children's Hospital."

"I should get one of those," I said. "I was born here too."

Cheryl laughed. "Aren't they wonderful? I keep them at arm's length to remind myself that our patients are so tiny."

"It must be overwhelming to realize that you are the leader of an institution where you began as a member of the nursing staff."

"Oh, it is," Cheryl, said, "but I don't really think about it a lot. I remember when I was first here; I wanted so badly to start a patient-advisory group to identify problem areas. When I returned as president, I was sitting in the chair one day and a light bulb went off. I can remember thinking, 'I'm the president, and I can do that now'." Cheryl laughs. "A lot of leadership is accomplished through communication, discipline, routine, communication forums, and meeting with staff members. The patient advisory groups and the parent advisory groups provide us with solid feedback that we can use to make the necessary improvements."

"Is it difficult to balance a strict discipline and routine here at the hospital, relative to your home life? When I was speaking with Dr. Caty, he mentioned that while he is a surgeon here, there isn't anyone handing him things at home."

Cheryl laughed. "And there's no one listening to my directions at home, either. Actually, the support of my family is instrumental to my work here. In this line of work, I've been asked to put in long hours. My husband and children were always so supportive. My parents, Richard and Catherine Kemp, were always there for us. There were so many days and nights when they watched our children."

Cheryl's pride flashed through as she spoke of each of her children. Erin is currently on-staff at the hospital as a member of the public relations team. Erin's presence at the hospital makes Cheryl extremely proud. "One day Erin called me to ask me to speak at an event in the Variety-8 playroom. I remember thinking that that's where she was born. It was wonderful."

"How about the challenges ahead?" I asked.

"There are plenty," Cheryl said. "First and foremost is keeping up with technology. We're also working on a new ambulatory building, and we want to continue to improve the facilities. Then there are the shortages of pharmacists and the shortage of nurses to deal with. Yet our number one task is to keep the energy level up."

"There are a number of units, departments, and staff members discussed in the book," I said. "My main frustration with writing the story is that I am unable to highlight the work of everyone here, but can you comment on a few of those departments?"

"Certainly."

"The PICU comes quickly to mind because that's where the bulk of Jake's care was done."

"It's a terrific unit with a strong medical staff and an equally strong nursing staff. I'm extremely proud of the work they do."

"Stone's Buddies," I said.

"It's a terrific program that is made stronger by the energy level of Joanne Lana. When I think of the work done for the families with terminally ill children, through the program, it makes me very proud."

"The NICU?"

"It's a beautiful unit with a dedicated staff of nurses. That's the very beginning of life, and there isn't anything more precious or valuable."

"It would probably be safe to say that you're proud of the efforts of your staff, right?"

"Of course, but as I tell the staff, good things don't just come to you; you have to earn them. If we do our job and take good care of our patients, the doctors will continue to trust us and send their patients to us. You know, some mornings, I may come into the hospital thinking of something else, like something that needs to be done at home, but when I walk through the lobby, the reason why I am here always comes back to me. I see the looks on the faces of the worried parents, or I may see a young, sick child. I know that we have a very important job to do, and just like the rest of the staff, I strive to do my job to the best of my abilities."

"So, you're proud to be here?" I asked, even though I already knew the answer.

"Absolutely," Cheryl said. "What happens here is truly special."

★   ★   ★

For the hundredth time, I headed down the hall and out toward the Hodge Street parking ramp. This was to be my final interview for the book, and I was a little sad knowing that my job was nearly complete. As I stepped outside, it occurred to me that Cheryl Klass was a remarkable leader working with a truly gifted staff of people. Yet, more than anything else, I understood that the Western New York Community and the people of Buffalo, New York were extremely fortunate to have the Women & Children's Hospital in their own backyard.

CHAPTER 22

The Story of Anthony Stinson
Part V

"Do what you can, with what you have, where you are."
—*Theodore Roosevelt*

"A mother is not a person to lean upon,
but a person to make leaning unnecessary."
—*Dorothy Canfield*

Upon meeting Anthony Stinson, I wrote the words, "There wasn't a single thing in my life that prepared me to meet Anthony Stinson."

After spending time with Trina Stinson, Anthony Stinson and Nicholas Stinson, I must say that there isn't a single thing in my life that quite prepared me to meet a family with more heart and courage. The Stinson family learned to face the most difficult of circumstances and not only survive, but flourish as a unit, with love, respect and honor serving as their guideposts.

It wasn't an easy transformation and there will be difficult battles ahead, but as I summarize the story of Anthony Stinson, as told in the loving voice of his adoring mother, I must admit that there have been few other people who have affected me in such a manner.

We neared the end of our interview at the Stinson home. Trina had been speaking for well over two hours, and I had been working hard to understand how anyone could handle such a difficult situation. As we spoke, Anthony lay prone in his crib, receiving loving touches and sweet caresses at the hand of his mother. Nicholas had been off and playing, but he certainly drifted closer to the living room, no doubt wondering why we had been speaking so long. Yet, there were still a few questions that needed to be answered.

"How do you do this day in and day out and still smile?" I asked finally.

Trina smiled sheepishly, as though she didn't deserve the respect that I had implied. She seemed to think about it for a split-second, but eventually she chose her very special words.

"My life has been devoted to keeping my children safe. I suppose that it would have been my life anyway, but it is definitely more pronounced. I just need to see Nicholas and Anthony happy. I ask God every night for the strength to make it work."

"God?" I asked. "When we spoke of God during the discussion of Anthony's illness, you had your doubts."

"It took a long time," Trina said as she sighed deeply. "As the years have gone by, I realize that God is with me. Although He has not allowed Anthony to recover, He gave me the love and strength to learn what I have in order to keep Anthony alive. He blessed me by giving me my family. He blessed me with an absolute darling of a son in Nicholas. I can't imagine what it would have been like if Nick hadn't been so caring, helpful, smart, and wise beyond his years."

Trina's voice had dropped in pitch, but I leaned closer to catch each and every word.

"He blessed me with a wonderful, loving mother who helps me in every way that she can. Since Anthony has been sick, she comes to my home twice a week to do our laundry. She buys clothes and shoes for the children, restocks Anthony's medical supplies, and keeps an eye on Nick while I'm taking Anthony to his doctor appointments, or the emergency room. My mother is a special, special woman who I love dearly, and God blessed me with her. I had to remember that. People have been wonderful. My Aunt Deborah and my Uncle Dennis have been absolutely irreplaceable. Ever since Anthony got sick, they have sent me money every other week. They have shown their love, and it taught me to believe again."

Trina was certainly emotional as she spoke of the love and support that she's received over the years. She has come full-circle in her relationship with God, but there are more reasons than her relationship with her giving family.

"God blessed me with wonderful nurses who help me take care of Anthony. It's so obvious to me that they have fallen in love with my boys. They are a part of my family now, and each has gone above and beyond for Anthony. I need to mention each of their names again," Trina says, and she recites the names with reverie as though she is reading the nominations for the Academy Award for Best Actor: Sarah Johnson LPN, Aimee Horan LPN, Deb Powers, RN, Lyn Baker RN, John Nashke LPN, and Shannon Flick LPN."

"Still, when you speak and think of God, it must have been a hell of a ride to go from what was total doubt to complete acceptance."

Trina nodded. "Of course, but when I was in doubt it was because I was dwelling on the negative. I can't even mention all that I am blessed with. Anthony's Special Education Teacher, Bonnie Sikes, helped me to realize that I had to count my blessings first. My God, so many people have helped me through this devastating journey that it would be real selfish of me if I didn't see them as blessings. I am just so grateful."

"Do you still grieve?" I asked.

"Of course," Trina answered quickly. "I grieve for the life we had so long ago. I envy the people who can take their children on vacations, to the playground, or an amusement park, or even to the grocery store. I envy the mothers who can watch their children play sports or just play outside and get mud in the house. I envy the children that can walk, talk, and play with their brother.

There are many, many things that people take for granted, and I want to beg them not to."

Trina spoke the words with conviction, and I realized it was because she had accepted them in her golden heart. She paused for a long moment before continuing. "Although we can't do a lot of the things other families do, we adapt to what we have. The three of us are always in Anthony's room and we listen to a lot of music together. This time of the year is the best because we listen to Christmas music. Our favorite is *Dominic the Italian Christmas Donkey.* It's pretty funny." Trina offered a wonderful smile. "Nick and I dance around and sometimes, if Anthony allows it, I take his arms and dance with him while he's in the bed or the wheelchair. Nick and I play games too, and we always try and include Anthony. I help Anthony with his decisions, and usually either he or Nick win. Somehow, I'm always on the losing end."

Trina was absolutely vibrant as she explained the fun that she has with the boys. I couldn't help but smile right along with her.

"Nick is a huge Sabres fan, so we'll watch the games too. Anthony is usually in bed, but once in awhile Nick helps me get Anthony out of his bed and into the wheelchair. Most of the time, the three of us just hang out with our dog Cora. We spend a lot of good times together."

Still, Trina's eyes grew moist as she thought about what might have been. Despite all of the fun that she has with her sons, she realized that there could be so much more.

"Anthony can't go outside when it's too cold or too hot. In fact, he can't go outside if it's too windy or too humid, either. We don't go out together much because Anthony needs someone beside him during transport in case he needs suctioning, has a seizure, or stops breathing. Sometimes in the summer, if the weather cooperates, we can go outside after dinner. Nick helps me put Anthony into the wheelchair and we'll go for a walk, or Nick and I will play catch, or basketball, or soccer. I do this thing with Anthony so that he feels as though he's dribbling the basketball and then throwing it."

"How do you do that?" I asked.

"I'll take his hand over the side of the wheelchair and use his hand to hit the ball so he's dribbling it. Then I take both of his hands and help him throw it. It's not easy because his arms are very heavy, but before too long when Nick saw how I did it, he started doing it for his brother. It makes me so proud to see how Nick helps his brother. In fact, I was going to get rid of the small basket that they used as Nick had certainly outgrown it, but he told me that he wanted to keep it because it's the perfect height for Anthony to make baskets out of his wheelchair."

"Nick has had to grow up faster than other children," I commented, "and yet, he's such a giving child."

"He's an amazing boy," Trina said. "The boys' birthdays are very close together, so we celebrate them together. Nick will open a present for himself and then, without being asked, he'll open one of Anthony's presents, take off the card and hold it close to his brother's face, and then read it to him. Then he'll take Anthony's present and show it to him. It's amazing that a child of eight would take the time for his brother. I know that if I were his age, I would be just ripping the paper off of my own presents."

"Do you realize what caring, loving children you are raising?" I asked.

"I'm really trying," Trina said. "I learned that I can't afford to be sad, angry or depressed all the time. What kind of life would it be for them if I constantly cried over what happened? Life is too short to waste by being miserable all the time, especially when the boys are depending on me."

"Trina, I know that I am speaking for everyone who has the chance to read this story when I say that you're an amazing person."

Trina waved me off and looked away. "The feeling of being depressed is not a feeling that I enjoy," she said. "There are definitely tough days, and I'm not always in the greatest of moods, but if I can make my children comfortable, I can get through anything."

Trina paused for a long while. She considered the long, difficult road that she had traveled, and true to her nature, she spoke of her gratitude for The Women & Children's Hospital of Buffalo.

"I get tremendous satisfaction in being on the Family-Centered Care Advisory Council. The hospital and the staff have saved Anthony's life on many occasions. When I think of the hospital, I think of the wonderful people. Chaplain Betty comes immediately to mind. Chaplain Betty always had time for me. She never made me feel rushed when we were talking. Chaplain Betty saw Anthony before he got sick and has been there to comfort me through the years. She comforted me when Anthony had his trach put in, in June of 2003. She was right there beside me again in August when Anthony started having tremors again. They were the same sort of tremors that he had in April of 2002, and I was sure that this time they would kill him. I was maniacal! I was begging the doctors for more Ativan, more seizure medications, anything! I was just so afraid the he would die. The doctors finally tried the Ketogenic Diet in an attempt to get the seizures to stop, but Anthony stopped breathing and had to go back to the PICU. That's where Chaplain Betty met me again. We talked about Anthony dying, and I didn't think that there was a chance that I could be calmed down, but Chaplain Betty comforted me."

Trina shook her head as though to clear her mind. I was so fascinated with her outlook on life that I felt as if I could listen to her speak of her children all night.

"I haven't been able to make Anthony better. I'm still working at it, though." Trina looked away from me to the crib. "I've accepted that this is the life that we have now, and I am going to do the best I can to make it okay for them. Through every difficult time in their lives, I will be there. When they are hurt or in trouble, I'll be there. When they are sad or lonely, I'll be there. And when they are happy or celebrating, I'll be there too. I'll help them along their way, you know?"

Trina had tears deep in her eyes, but she was comfortable allowing them to stay right there.

"I let them know that no matter what, I love them unconditionally. No matter what, I will always be there for them. I will try to help them fix their problems. I will allow them the chance to cope with pain. I tried to protect and shield them from ever being hurt, but sometimes life doesn't allow a mother to do that."

I felt a sharp pain just behind my own eyes and I understood that, if I didn't end the interview soon, I was going to blubber all over the Stinson family. I struggled for a breath of air just as Nicholas entered the room.

"Hey, Mom," he said, "can I watch television with Anthony?"

Trina hopped down off the hospital bed. She lowered the rail and tousled Nick's hair as he moved past her and snuggled on the bed next to his little brother. It was all the beauty that I could take and I thought to myself that I couldn't handle anymore. I glanced at the scene once more and watched as Nick placed his hand on his brother's leg. Anthony didn't respond, of course, but Nick didn't seem to mind. He touched his brother's skin softly, and I was allowed to see and feel the love. Now I said what I was feeling. "Okay, that's enough," I whispered, and Trina laughed because she knew what I was feeling.

As I gathered my notebooks and headed to the car, I opened the door to a beautiful fall night. Trina followed me out the front door. I walked away, not knowing if there was anything I could say to summarize one of the most beautiful, devastating, heartwarming, confusing nights of my life. I realized that this was Trina's life. I understood she was more courageous than anyone I have ever met. Slowly, with those tears burning my eyes, I turned to Trina who was waiting at the door. "I need to write the story of you and your boys," I said.

"If you could do that." Trina's voice faded to a whisper. I didn't hear what else she had to say. I didn't need to.

★   ★   ★

A couple of months later, I received an e-mail from Trina. I present it as it appeared on my computer screen.

"Over the summer, I was cleaning out my closets and I found the poem that woman gave me three-and-a-half years ago at Anthony's benefit. I understand it better now and I've hung it on the wall in my living room."

Anthony's Special Mother

Most women become mothers by accident, some by choice, a few by social pressures, and a couple by habit. This year nearly 100,000 women will become mothers of special needs children. Did you ever wonder how mothers of special needs children are chosen?

Somehow, I visualize God hovering over earth, selecting his instruments for propagation with great care and deliberation. As He observes, He instructs His angels to make notes on a giant ledger.

"Armstrong, Beth…son. Patron Saint, Matthew."

"Forest, Marjorie…daughter. Patron Saint, Cecilia."

"Rutledge, Carrie…twins. Patron Saint…give her Gerald. He's used to profanity."

Finally, He passes Trina's name to an angel and smiles, "Give Trina a special needs child."

The angel is curious. "Why this one, God? She is so happy."

"Exactly," smiles God. "Could I give a special needs child a mother who does not know laughter? That would be cruel."

"But does she have patience?" Asks the angel.

"I don't want her to have too much patience, or she will drown in a sea of self-pity and despair. Once the shock and resentment wear off, she'll handle it. I watched her today. She has that sense of self and independence that are so rare and so necessary in a mother. You see, Anthony has his own world. She has to make him live in this world, and that's not going to be easy."

"But Lord, I don't even think she believes in you."

God smiles. "No matter, I can fix that. This one is perfect. She has just enough selfishness."

The angel gasps, "Selfishness? Is that a virtue?"

God nods. "If she can't separate herself from her child occasionally, she'll never survive. Yes, here is a woman whom I will bless with a child less than perfect. She doesn't realize it yet, but she is to be envied."

"She will never take for granted a spoken word. She will never consider a step ordinary. When her child says 'Mommy' for the first time, she will be witness to a miracle and know it. When she describes a tree or a sunset to her blind child, she will see it as few people ever see my creations."

"I will permit her to see the things I see—ignorance, cruelty, and prejudice—and allow her to rise above them. She will never be alone. I will be at her side, every minute of every day of her life. She is doing my work, as surely as she is here by my side."

"And what about Trina's patron Saint?" Asks the angel, his pen poised in mid-air.

God smiles. "A mirror will suffice."

Trina wrote: "Cliff, it took me a long time to get to where I am today. I have learned so many things along the way, and you truly don't realize the capacity for love and strength that you have inside of you until you are forced to use it. I hope that this can help people understand that you should *never* take your children for granted! Show them each and every day that you love them, no matter what. Be thankful that they can play, or even fight with their siblings, or that they can fall and scrape a knee, or are able to be put in time out…I know that these are frustrating to parents, but *trust me*, I long for them daily."

CHAPTER 23

The Story of the Fazzolari Family

"The potential possibilities of any child
are the most intriguing and stimulating in all creation."
—Ray L. Wilbur

During the writing of these stories, the Fazzolari family celebrated the five-year anniversary of Jake's release from The Women & Children's Hospital of Buffalo. The annual celebration of Jake's successful surgery is a widely anticipated day for the family. In fact, November 5th of each year is referred to as Family Day. It is simply a day spent in appreciation of one another's company. It is a day to thank God for our blessings. It is a day that falls within three weeks of Thanksgiving, but it is our day to spend together, pure and simple.

In 2001, the Fazzolari family suffered through the diagnosis of a massive tumor in the center of Jake's chest. At the time of this discovery, Jake was just four years old. Over the course of eight tension-filled weeks, our lives were turned upside down. As a family, we worked closely with the hospital staff. Jake underwent chemotherapy treatments in an effort to shrink the massive tumor so that the surgeons could do their work. Jake's hair fell out; I shaved my own head in an effort to make him feel comfortable, and the tumor did not shrink. Jake's hair grew back; mine did not.

Through the very anxious days, our family faced some of life's most perplexing questions. We leaned heavily on a strong faith, and a most cooperative staff of doctors and nurses. Jake and I watched one cartoon after another, and I battled nightmares that showed Frosty the Snowman melting in the greenhouse.

In the end, a well-thought-out treatment plan, and the steady hands of the talented surgeons, allowed us the opportunity to return home with a healthy child. We were counting on a miracle, and while there was so much that we did not know, the men and women who worked on Jake were unbelievably passionate about providing the very best of care.

Appreciation is a strong emotion. It shows up in our dreams, in our memory banks, and occasionally right there when we are speaking with the person who deserves the praise. I have certainly appreciated the time and effort of the people interviewed for this compilation of stories. There are some mornings when my heart beats faster as I consider some of the sacrifices made by the men and women who work hour after hour at The Women & Children's Hospital of Buffalo. I began this little journey firmly believing that those chronicled in this work deserve to be recognized and praised. I ended the story with the realization that it truly doesn't matter one way or another to any one of them. There are hundreds of people working in the hospital who are not looking for praise. To be sure, each of the individuals chosen for this story weren't the least bit interested in any of my praise. Rather, these unique individuals had the singular goal of being better in their chosen profession.

There were certainly moments during the writing of the story when I felt some of the same frustrations expressed by some of the men and women who were interviewed. It is unbelievably distressing to me that there are too many people in this country who have no idea how they would pay for the care necessary if their children were sick. The Women and Children's Hospital of Buffalo's policy of treating all, without regard, strengthens my faith in humanity.

A troubling frustration of mine that is borne of the inability of society to accept the true heroes of the community was quickly dismissed by all of those involved in healthcare. Every single year

I am annoyed by a pampered athlete who fails to appreciate the fact that he is paid a king's ransom for catching a ball, while a dedicated nurse or doctor is held up for public ridicule if they make even a single mistake. True to the grace of each person interviewed, being accepted as a hero was not a consideration.

Yet that is not to say that all is perfect. The Family-Centered Care initiative at the hospital is proof enough that things can be done even better. It is disconcerting to realize that there must be an initiative to work with compassion and respect. But, those reading along should understand that healthcare is not a perfect science. In fact, in recent years, it is painfully apparent that the United States of America is slipping on the world stage in the very treatment of their citizens. The Women & Children's Hospital of Buffalo, to its credit, continues to strive to be better.

The lack of funds to implement the necessary programs is also difficult to comprehend, but again the Western New York community continues to rally behind the hospital on an annual basis, and once more, that is cause for celebration. Perhaps it would be easier to live in a society where a hospital didn't have to campaign for the dollars needed to sustain itself, but I learned early on in my writing career that ideals and norms aren't easily addressed.

On Family Day in the Fazzolari household, we give thanks to the people who worked with us at the hospital. The names of those who were critical to the care of our son rush back to us in a flood of emotion. Once more, I offer the acknowledgement that was included in *Counting on a Miracle*:

As a family we thank Doctor Marc Levitt, Doctor Michael Caty, Doctor Joy Graf, Pediatric Nurse Practitioner Karen Iacono, Doctor Doron Feldman, Doctor Bradley Fuhrman, Doctor James Foster, and OR Nurses Rosemary Silvashy, Helen Noblett, and Patricia Long and the entire staff of physicians and technicians that saved Jake's life. Special thanks to the ICU staff, including, but not limited to, Jeff Klempf, Ken Smith, and Ellen Eckhardt. Thanks to Janine and Neal Cross for years of friendship and talking us through it. To Sue Mazurchuk, Jake's all-time favorite nurse—you're a special person. A hearty thanks to photographer Brian Smistek for his outstanding work.

I offer sincere appreciation to Nurse Kathy Humphrey, Dr. Yi Horng Lee, Dr. Omar S. Al-Ibrahim, Nursing Supervisor Sharon Hewson, Nurse Manager Judy Murko (see you in church), Chief Nursing Officer LuAnn Brown, and to Mary Ellen Creighton, the Director of Pediatric Nursing. Finally, to John Moscato, who had to field about a hundred of my calls and e-mails. John was not only undeniably professional and helpful, he's also a great guy to talk to, and that's a true gift.

I would also like to acknowledge the strength and courage shown by the parents in the stories of Anthony Stinson, Alexia Grace Kilroy and Olivia Stockmeyer. It was a true pleasure to work with Kevin and Kim Stockmeyer, Mark and Brooke Kilroy and Trina Stinson. Writing is a very solitary experience that is dependent upon a voice that people want to hear. I was blessed to be able to add the voices of Kim, Kevin, Mark, Brooke and Trina. They are truly classy individuals who deserve praise for allowing their stories to be out there for all. It is very easy to compartmentalize, and to feel sympathy for families who have sick children. It is even easier to appreciate that your own children are healthy, but the true testament of the strength of a human being is the ability to see beyond their own situation and to offer some assistance.

I also need to thank Olivia Stockmeyer, Taylor Adamo, Alexia Grace Kilroy, Anthony Stinson and Nicholas Stinson. Above all else, this is a story of and about children. I can't begin to explain the love that I feel for the children who have endured and will continue to endure the most difficult of challenges. I pray for each of you every day.

A special thank-you is extended to Jill Kelly and the Kelly family. Hunter Kelly's life is a testament to love, devotion, and dedication. It is difficult to put into words how appreciative I am of Jill's participation in this project. Simply stated, her love for her children, and her tremendous understanding of faith, inspired me to keep writing.

Finally, I offer my thanks to my own family. Without you, Family Day would not exist. To my wife, Kathy, I see my stories in your eyes. Your support is unbelievable, even when I throw the whole weekend schedule off by being alone with the computer. To my sons, Matthew, Jake and Sam: Daddy loves you.

The Rocking Chair by Ellen Eckhardt, PICU Nurse

"I've learned that people will forget what you said,
people will forget what you did,
but people will never forget how you made them feel."
—*Maya Angelou*

The rain was spilling out of the sky and
the candle's flame was soft.
The white of the piano keys were highlighted by the candlelight.
There was stillness in the air.
I am a rocker, whose life has been very full;
full of each and every person and their happiness or woes;
each person who took a moment to find solace in my presence.

As I glide back and forth,
I drift into the memory of each and every life that has been
touched by my just being there.

There was the night a new baby was born…
many, many years ago. It was very much like tonight,
only the candlelight was truly the only available light.
I remember moving forward, then back, then forward,
then back, as a woman sang lullabies
to a precious, sleeping baby.

Then there was the day that a curious toddler
took great efforts to sit on my lap.
The giggles, as I wiggled back and forth,
made the sunshine coming through the window seems so
much brighter that day.

I was the landing for a game of hide'n'seek.
Boy, did I wobble that day!

I was a spectator at the Sunday football games.
The big, soft cushions of the couch and
the reclining of the lounge chair were, by far,
more appealing on those lazy days.

I jumped at the chance to be part of a bedtime story hour.
The quest to understand in those innocent, sparkly eyes made
the anticipation of each new story so worthwhile.

Those concert nights ended with pictures of me
and the star of the show.

The very next day could be the day my lap
got soaked with grape juice.
I figured I was changed forever, but somehow,
most of it came out.
Everyone says that the part that is left is
the most beautiful part of my cushion.
Imagine that.

One day I was very much part of the anticipation of a first date.
Since he was five minutes late,
the half hour of rocking turned into thirty-five minutes.

The day of their wedding a few years later,
I was the center of the four generation picture.
Oh, the tears that day.

It seemed like I was used more and more after that.
The rocking was peaceful, or, well…
yes, there were the days I was part of the corner thinking spot
after an argument.

Then one day it seemed the house was quieter.
The devoted family dog was still at my feet.
I sensed a loss. A great loss.
The lullabies that had been sung became quiet songs
of memories. For that was all she had.
He died in his sleep, as she hoped she would some day.
I felt absolutely helpless.
Her empty heart echoed her sadness as a tear would land
on my arm now and then.
Somehow though, the more she rocked, the better I felt…
and I think she did too.

I became a haven for reading: comedies, biographies,
the daily newspaper or cards from loved ones.
Before going to bed at night, she opened her bible and read it,
a new verse every night.
I learned a lot.

A day came when there was a beautiful breeze
and the sun came shining in on my faded grape juice spot.
The family dog and I shared some quiet moments,
as I wondered where she was.
I realized, as they took me out the door,
that time marches on.
Now, I'm going to a new home, to learn more about life.

Heaven's Blanket
by Ellen Eckhardt,
PICU Nurse

Misty came home from school with a far-off look in her eyes.

"What's on your mind, honey?" her mother asked.

"Mom, where do we go when we die? I mean, we're here, then we die, and we go to heaven. Well, I just don't understand. I can't imagine what it will really be like."

"What made you think of this today?"

"Kristen's cousin Hope just died. She was really sick and had been in the hospital, but it seemed like she was getting better. Then she died suddenly. Kristen's so sad and I wish I could make her feel better."

"Come on, Misty. Let's go for a walk, you 'n me."

The winter snow was beautiful, light, fluffy, and crystal-like in the sunshine.

"See how pure the snow looks, so untouched and perfect?" Misty's mother began. "Though we will be finished with our life on earth, we will be in a different dimension of life. We will be living that life, and the peace will be a peace that we only dream of having here."

"But will Kristen ever see her cousin again?" Misty asked.

"Not here, but yes, she will. It will be in a different dimension, in a way that goes beyond our earthly connection with one another. They will connect on a spiritual level."

"What do you mean, Mom?"

"We know that we are living life for a purpose, each and every one of us. We know how we'd like to communicate with others, but so often we fall short, and that's human nature."

Misty brightened up. "Once we die, we'll be able to take on that challenge?"

"Live in perfect harmony and always get along." Misty's mom smiled as she picked up a handful of fluffy snow. "We will experience no pain, and we'll be filled with love, forever. Yes, however, it won't be a challenge, but a gift. It will just be."

"How?" Misty asked.

"Look at the shimmering snow crystals. They are millions of flakes that turn into a beautiful blanket, covering a dimension of life: the grass. The grass is beautiful in the mid-summer when the rain has nourished it and the sun has helped it grow. But sometimes it becomes brittle and brown without the rain and sun, kind of like us here on earth. When we don't recognize the love that is around us…everywhere, every day…and we don't let it soak into our hearts, we become weak and vulnerable. As the summer turns to autumn, and autumn to winter, it becomes sad to think of losing the summer beauty and to accept the heavy winter snow's burden on our spirits. That is how death seems to appear. There is that great pain of missing a part of ourselves when we lose a relative or a friend. The beautiful part of it is that what is seemingly a heavy burden is a blanket of beauty in heaven. It's one that is made of millions of people who were a part of life on earth. Just like the snowflakes, each person is different in little ways, or big ways, and they all come together to make an incredible blanket. The shining flakes perfect the snow into something mystical. A cold, white covering is transformed into a shimmering, warm site that is a lasting beauty in heaven."

"How can that help lessen the pain we feel when someone we love dies?" Misty's blue eyes sparkled in the sunshine as she gazed innocently into her mother's eyes.

"The best thing to learn is that just as we are standing here, experiencing the beauty of the shining snow, we can try to spread more love here. Though we will never have the perfection of heaven here on earth, we can try and tap into the feeling it gives us to be loved by our friend, or relative, and we can spread that love to someone else. Each bit of love that we were given, that we pass onto someone else, will help us shed our sadness. That's because when love is given away, it fills us with a special feeling. Then when we die, we will all be like a snowflake that falls down on the shimmering blanket, becoming part of the eternal beauty, which is heaven."

"That's when the love of our best friends will shine down on us forever, Mom?"

"That's right, Misty. We have to let God be our friend here, too. Though life isn't always easy, we have a friend who walks with us every second of every day. All we have to do is remember that God is there, and we have to thank Him for taking the worst of the pain away."

"Mom, I love you," Misty said, as she wrapped her arms around her mother.

"I love you too, Misty."

The next day, as she walked into school, Misty glanced at the sky. She noticed the distinct outline of the puffy white clouds against the radiant blue background. *Every day, the sky is the home of clouds, expressing themselves in different ways. And it's because of these clouds that we enjoy this snowy blanket.*

Misty turned to see a section of untouched, glistening snow between the fence outlining the vast schoolyard and the entrance she was about to proceed through. A contented sigh accompanied her, as she remembered that school was about to start.

As Misty closed her locker, she noticed Kristen's approach.

"Hey, Misty."

"Hi, Kristen," Misty said with a smile. "How are you?"

"Good. Actually, I feel better today."

"I'm glad. Why?"

"Well, when I got home from school yesterday, I went out-side to make a snow fort with Andrew. We were trying to pack the snow, but it was so fluffy that it would have taken the rest of the winter to get enough packed for our fort. We decided to make angels in the snow, instead."

"That's cool," Misty said. "My mom and I went for a walk in all that fluff. It seemed like the snow was especially pretty. It sparkled."

"I know," Kristen said. "The deep snow was so light and fluffy that it started to cover me and my angel as I started to make her wings. The sun was shining over me, making each snowflake sparkle. For the first time since Hope died, I thought about how nice it must be in heaven."

Misty felt a warm tingle inside. "You were being covered by a blanket of snow, weren't you?"

"I guess you could call it that, yeah." Kristen shrugged her shoulders and smiled a crooked smile. "I felt like Hope was right there with me. I can't really explain it."

"I'm sure she was, Kristen. I'm sure she was."

Misty put her arm around her friend as they headed to the classroom to start their day.

Note from Ellen Eckhardt: Dedicated to my dad, Lester Eckhardt, who passed away on February 7, 2007…and to Hunter Kelly, who passed away on August 5, 2005. Dad, at the age of 80, and Hunter, at the age of 8, showed me the true meaning of strength.

To My Co-workers
by Ellen Eckhardt,
PICU Nurse

*"Each and every person I meet has something to teach me…
if I only open my eyes to see,"*
—Ellen Eckhardt

"As I reflect on the last twenty-three years of my career at The Women & Children's Hospital of Buffalo, my heart goes in many directions. First and foremost, though, I reflect on the people that I've met along the way. The people who have taught me what it means to care, and to keep on caring, even when it seems that there is every reason to throw in the towel. Exhaustion, frustration, sadness, anger, confusion, and questioning are all very real. Every day I have stepped into our hospital, though, I believe I have become a better person, and that is because of each and every person in our working family. The exhaustion turns to renewed energy as I feel the energy around me. The frustration turns to determination as I feel the forward motion of medicine today. The sadness turns to inner peace, as I realize that we all have a small part in making this better in any way that we can. The anger turns to contentment when I focus on the team effort and realize how negativity can be contagious. The confusion turns to clarity when I notice how each person's piece in this complex puzzle is critical to the final masterpiece. The questioning turns to trust in God's bigger plan, that is forever unfolding. And the one that can be all-consuming—the bitterness—turns into acceptance. We are human and we have our limitations. What challenges our limitations, however, is forward vision—a vision in working together to make change happen. That can only happen with a cohesive team effort, and I feel as though I am part of an absolutely incredible team. I am proud to say that I work at The Women & Children's Hospital of Buffalo. To each of my co-workers, I say thank you. Thank you for teaching me endurance. Thank you for teaching me excellence. Thank you for teaching me critical thinking. Most of all, thank you for teaching me to love when it hurts. We have such a privilege, to learn from our children, and from each other. I believe that the strength we have as a working family extends to our community and beyond. We can never underestimate what may happen tomorrow, because of how we worked together today.

A special thank-you to Cheryl Klass, who was my head nurse when I began work at the hospital. You were a great role model then, and you continue to be one now. How fortunate we are to have you in the forefront, as our president.

The Women & Children's Hospital of Buffalo

Since its founding in 1892, The Women & Children's Hospital of Buffalo has been devoted to providing the ultimate in pediatric and maternal health care. As a regional referral center and one of only three pediatric hospitals in the United States with a maternity unit, WCHOB provides unique patient care to the eight-county Western New York area.

The hospital serves more than 28,000 inpatients annually, and more than 150,000 outpatients visit the emergency department or one of the 45 specialty clinics each year. Virtually all medical and surgical problems of infants, children, and adolescents are available for resident education programs.

WCHOB has a long history of commitment to tertiary and primary care pediatrics. Associated with this commitment, the hospital also has a history of innovative research, much of which has practical applications that measurably improve the quality of life of children. Past and ongoing efforts include:

- The development of the Guthrie screening test for PKU.
- Clinical testing of exogenous calf lung surfactant in premature infants.
- First clinical trials with nitric oxide ventilation.
- First studies of the use of liquid ventilation for pulmonary oxygen delivery.
- Use of ECMO in the care of critically ill children.

The hospital offers a wide range of advanced care, from its designated Level 3 regional intensive care nursery staffed by a dedicated transport team, respiratory therapists, and specially trained nurses—to its division of maternal-fetal medicine, which treats patients before they are born. The hospital also offers

extensive outpatient care, including genetic diagnostic and coun-
seling services, chronic disease clinics, child and adolescent psy-
chiatric services, and a world-renowned rehabilitation clinic.

Included in the hospital's 313 beds are 67 maternity beds. Its
maternity and high-risk maternity programs are complemented
by its intensive care nursery, which cares for nearly 1,000 critically
ill full-term and premature newborns annually, many of them
weighing as little as one to two pounds. WCHOB has one of the
highest rates of survival for premature neonates in the country.

A private, non-profit hospital, Women & Children's Hospital
is the major teaching affiliate of the State University of New York
at Buffalo (SUNY) School of Medicine and Biomedical Sciences'
Department of pediatrics. The University's Department of
Obstetrics and Gynecology is housed here as well. More than 700
medical, nursing, and allied health students study here each year.
As part of its commitment to primary care, WCHOB maintains
two clinics in underserved areas. In addition, a commitment has
been made to be intimately involved in providing primary care to
school-based clinics.

Located in a beautiful residential section of central Buffalo,
among streets lined with majestic Victorian mansions and stately
oaks, the hospital campus is easily accessible by private or public
transportation, including Buffalo's light rail rapid transit line that
runs from the downtown area to the University's South Campus, where the medical school is located.

The University's medical school has over 2,000 faculty members, more than 300 of whom are full-time. House officers in
pediatrics receive clinical faculty appointments in the University
and play a major role in teaching medical students. Because of
their faculty appointments, residents have access to the educa-
tional, cultural, and recreational facilities of the University.

For more information, please visit The Women & Children's
Hospital of Buffalo Home Page at www.wchob.org

To make a donation to the Women & Children's Hospital of
Buffalo, New York, contact: The Children's Hospital of Buffalo
Foundation: 219 Bryant Street, Buffalo, New York 14222-2099.